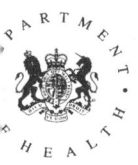

CW01510661

Negotiating in the Community

The Implications of Research Findings on Community Based Practice for the Implementation of the Community Care and Children Acts

Gerald Smale • Graham Tuson
Bandana Ahmad • Giles Darvill
Lynette Domoney • Eric Sainsbury

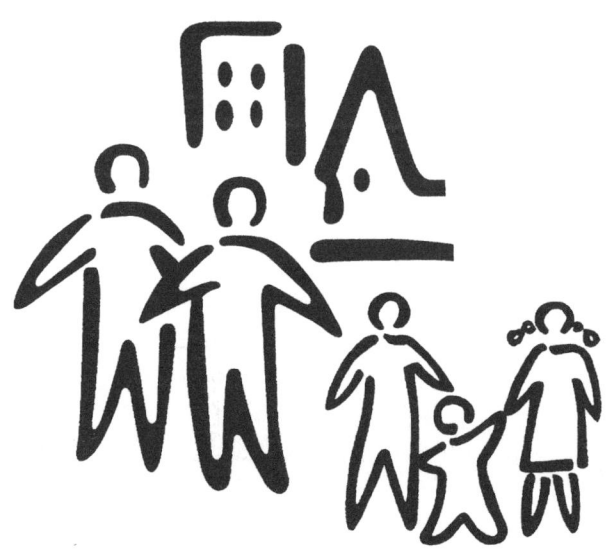

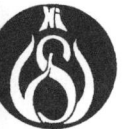

Practice and Development Exchange

National Institute for Social Work

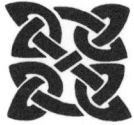

London: HMSO

ISBN 0 11 321666 1

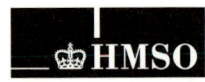

HMSO publications are available from:

HMSO Publications Centre
(Mail, fax and telephone orders only)
PO Box 276, London, SW8 5DT
Telephone orders 071-873 9090
General enquiries 071-873 0011
(queuing system in operation for both numbers)
Fax orders 071-873 8200

HMSO Bookshops
49 High Holborn, London, WC1V 6HB
071-873 0011 Fax 071-873 8200 (counter service only)
258 Broad Street, Birmingham, B1 2HE
021-643 3740 Fax 021-643 6510
33 Wine Street, Bristol, BS1 2BQ
0272 264306 Fax 0272 294515
9-21 Princess Street, Manchester, M60 8AS
061-834 7201 Fax 061-833 0634
16 Arthur Street, Belfast, BT1 4GD
0232 238451 Fax 0232 235401
71 Lothian Road, Edinburgh, EH3 9AZ
031-228 4181 Fax 031-229 2734

HMSO's Accredited Agents
(see Yellow Pages)

and through good booksellers

£7.50 net

This book is dedicated to Roy Pearson in memory of his commitment to improving practice and management in the personal Social Services

Contents

Preface

This work was commissioned by the Department of Health Social Services Inspectorate. The aim of the project was to identify how the literature informs the implementation of the NHS and Community Care and the Children Acts.

The literature to be reviewed included the work of the following:

Philip Abrams, Martin Bulmer and associates on Social Networks and Neighbourhood Care

Michael Bayley and associates on the Dinnington project

The Community Social Work Exchange publications of Practice and Development Exchange: National Institute for Social Work

Jane Gibbons' work on Family Support and Prevention

Roger Hadley and associates on Normanton and East Sussex

The work of David Challis and associates on the Kent Community Care Scheme

NISW Research Unit publications, particularly the Networks and Schemes projects and subsequent development work

Work of the Race Equality Unit based at NISW

The Self-Help Alliance evaluation material.

This report was completed in parallel with a companion volume: *Empowerment, Assessment, Care Management and the Skilled Worker* by Gerald Smale and Graham Tuson with Nina Biehal and Peter Marsh (Smale et al, 1993). The two publications should be read together.

Sir Roy Griffiths said that the aim of his *Agenda for Action* must be:

" ... to provide the structure and resources to support the initiatives, the innovation and the commitment at local level and to allow them to flourish; to encourage the success stories in one area to become the commonplace of achievement everywhere else. To prescribe from the centre will be to shrivel the pattern of local activity". (Griffiths, 1988 p.iv)

This review is presented in the spirit of this statement. Those planning and carrying out the implementation of the Children and NHS and Community Care Acts should take into consideration the lessons that can be learnt from recent past experience, particularly from those practitioners and managers whose practices and approach to service delivery have anticipated the Acts and their underlying principles.

Much has been said about the scope of the changes taking place in social work and social services and sometimes this gives the erroneous impression that the whole enterprise has to be reinvented. The research and development work reviewed here illustrates the progress that has been made in developing partnerships with members of the community to broaden the range of resources available to them, to widen their choices, and to strengthen their participation in the work of the services. The Griffiths report was explicit in relating the proposed reforms to developments in community based practice, pointing out that:

> "The recommendations as to the changed role for social services authorities were foreshadowed by the Barclay report in 1983. The essence of the present proposals is that there is machinery to ensure that it happens." (Griffiths, 1988 p.vii)

Sir Roy Griffiths has also drawn attention to the relevance of the work reviewed here, writing of the Dinnington project:

> "This project, while unique in the particular challenges encountered, has valuable lessons in terms of approach that can be usefully studied by those involved in the difficult, complex, and rewarding business of delivering services to people. I commend this report to all those interested in translating the rhetoric of community care into action." (Griffiths, 1988b p.ix)

The fact is that the bulk of care in the community is carried out by citizens and that professional services and intervention are peripheral activities. This leads to the fundamental assumption that community care for adults and the care and protection of children should be based on the care that already exists in the community. Workers should proceed through partnerships between the citizens involved in such care and those who provide services from either the public, voluntary or private sectors.

These assumptions were clearly identified by Barclay, are common to both the Community Care and Children Acts and have underpinned the approach to practice adopted by many of the practitioners and managers who participated in the research and development work reviewed.

Our particular concern was to identify the relationship between research findings and development experience and the underlying common principles of the Acts, rather than engage in a detailed discussion of the different interpretations of issues such as "care management." These common elements have been identified in a DoH discussion paper *Caring for People and the Children Act: Similarity and Differences* (1990). Using this as a baseline the research has been reviewed to identify the management and practice implications for operating on them. We have inevitably a particular perspective and set of values and hope they are clear to the reader.

The work reviewed was carried out in different settings using a range of methodologies and addressing different questions, but there is a significant degree of consistency in the major implications. Community care and child protection built on partnerships between professionals and citizens and designed to keep people in their own homes, match services to users' wishes and needs through collaboration between them, public, voluntary and other professional organisations, is not a simple, straightforward enterprise. No simple straightforward set of messages emerges from the literature that can be set against the Community Care and Children Acts guidelines.

We are confronted by a matrix of overlapping practice and management implications and many gaps in our knowledge where there is no sound evidence to guide practice. Continued research and development is of paramount importance if we are to have any idea of the impact of these reforms and be confident that people do have more control over their improving services.

The scope of the review

This review was not intended to be a comprehensive analysis of all research on community care for adults, services for children and child protection. Nor were we asked to tackle the extensive task of reviewing research that is relevant to all the areas of management and practice that the Acts cover. Both exercises would have required considerably more resources than those available for this project. The research, and so this review, does not address all aspects of the reforms. For example, none of the research reviewed evaluated complaints procedures nor, to our knowledge, social services departments that had such procedures in place. However, many of the managers and workers involved in the development activities had engaged in some work on setting up consultative arrangements with users, local people and other agencies that were a channel for complaints about services delivered as well as policy decisions about priorities. There are, then, significant issues in both Acts that are not touched on by this review.

The approach agreed with the DoH was to set up a working group to carry out a review of the literature. In addition the authors of the major reports were invited to participate in a series of forums to discuss the review and contribute to identifying the lessons for the new legislation. The proceedings of these discussions were recorded and analysed for the final report.

Wider consultations, with for example representatives of user groups or service providers, were not possible within the resources available. We are also acutely conscious of the fact that we were not able to do justice to much research that has valuable lessons for the implementation of these two Acts.

Working group members

Gerald Smale, Director, Practice and Development Exchange: National Institute for Social Work

Bandana Ahmad, Director, Race Equality Unit

Giles Darvill, Community Resources Management

Lynette Domoney, Information Development Officer, Practice and Development Exchange: National Institute for Social Work

Professor Eric Sainsbury, University of Sheffield

Graham Tuson, University of Southampton

Roy Pearson, Social Services Inspectorate: Department of Health.

Structure of the report

The report opens with an Executive Summary based on the discussion that takes place in Chapter Three: Implications of the Research for Management and Practice. References in this Section have been kept to a minimum. The research findings are reported more systematically in Chapter Two: Synthesis of the Research Findings.

Chapter Three examined the official guidelines for implementation of the new legislation then available in order to identify a core group of common operational principles. These were used to assist recognition of research findings relevant to implementation of the Acts.

Acknowledgments

This work was commissioned and supported by the Department of Health. We want to thank Roy Pearson for his contributions to discussions, encouragement, and essential advice. We are particularly grateful to the authors who gave their time and expertise and commented on an early draft of the report: Michael Bayley, David Challis, Michael Cooper, David Crosbie, Professor Roger Hadley, Professor Ian Sinclair, Ann Vickery, Michael Wardle. The conclusions presented here are those of the group writing this report and are not necessarily those of the DoH or SSI. This work could not have been completed without the skill, expertise and patience in the face of unreasonable demands of Nancy Dunlop, Nnennaya Onyekwere and Ann Vandersypen.

Chapter One
Executive Summary

Introduction

1.1 It is important to keep in mind the scale of "normal" care in the community as the essential context of service provision. For many dependent people (though not for all), the formal services are peripheral to their wellbeing. There are about 3.7 million "care managers" in Great Britain, none of whom are employed to care by social services departments, or anybody else. This excludes those who manage the care of their children.

1.2 Much of the research and development work reviewed here was carried out with practitioners and managers who shared at least some of the major assumptions that underpin the reforms. Their experience is relevant; care in the community does not have to be reinvented even though much of it has to be renegotiated with major participants.

The focus of professional services and intervention

1.3 The social situation is the appropriate unit of assessment. This includes the local and cultural expectations about "normal" patterns of care and support, the "clients'" and the "carers'" perceptions of their needs and of the resources available, the judgments of professionals and the nature of existing relationships. All are factors integral to any future "package of care" drawn from a combination of people's personal networks, available voluntary and professional services.

1.4 Most people enter residential care because of their social circumstances. Personal relationships are more significant indicators of the need for services than individual characteristics.

1.5 Social services professionals will have to act as agents of change as well as gatekeepers of resources. Their roles can be reformulated to fulfil the bridging functions necessary to develop, and provide choice from a coherent set of options.

1.6   Efforts to reform practice and management could be undermined by the basic assumptions that persist about the nature of care in the community. We have to confront the constant tendency to **regress to the individualisation of social problems.**

1.7   Social problems are the malfunctioning of a network of people: being old is not a serious problem any more than being a baby is one. Being either, without having appropriate relationships with others is, however, a "social problem".

General comments on the process of change

1.8   Many senior managers are reorganising their departments as a prime means of implementing the legislation in the absence of any other strategy for achieving change, and so the intention of the reforms "to support the initiative, the innovation and the commitment at the local level and to allow them to flourish", is in serious danger of being pushed aside. There is an urgent need to develop a greater understanding of the processes and management of innovation in planning, social work practice and service delivery because **how** change is implemented is crucial.

1.9   There can be no universal blueprints for services if consumers are to be involved in their planning and given more choice.

1.10   Changes in practice and attitudes take place over years not months and should be accompanied by organisational change. Wholesale reorganisations use up enormous amounts of energy and resources and may demoralise and sidetrack workers and management rather than help them to develop practice and services.

"Informal" care and the statutory services: the need to develop resources

1.11   It is naive to assume the "natural" existence of wider networks that can be called upon to meet people's needs without resources being put in to change the way people and organisations are currently relating to each other and to develop the potential for more care and appropriate control in the community.

1.12   Social networks are not simply sources of support. They are also
        sources of conflict, and the location of "social problems": enabling
        "normal" care to take place often requires a change in the way
        people relate to each other in their social networks and not just
        the delivery of a service. Social networks are diverse and in this
        lies their strength and relevance. It is crucial that managers and
        practitioners engage in work at the local level to develop
        resources and to expand options for care in the community for all
        age groups. There is a need to recognise that social services
        professionals are required to act as agents of change as well as
        resource brokers and deliverers of service.

1.13   Staff time needs to be explicitly allocated to development
        activities within the community. This is most likely to be
        available and effective if specialist staff are appointed within
        geographically located teams who can collectively maximise
        essential local knowledge.

Black and ethnic minority communities: exemplars of care and the need for changed relationships with service providers

1.14   There is much to be learnt from the way that black and ethnic
        minority groups have developed alternative forms of community
        care. It is necessary to develop partnerships between these
        resources and professional services, to overcome the barriers that
        have often led to people from minority groups not receiving the
        services they are entitled to.

Assessment and care management: one process, two activities?

1.15   Inevitably, conflict often exists between the demands and needs of
        referrers, carers and dependent people; between the different
        "users" of services, and between other people in the "client's"
        family and wider network.

1.16   Undertaking assessments and care management has to be
        negotiated within these conflicting needs, attitudes,
        expectations; as have definitions of the "problem", and its
        "solutions", to arrive at, and maintain, a workable and good
        enough package of care, as defined by users.

1.17   Services sensitive to the particular needs of people from all ethnic and other social groups will require workers to develop communication skills and a repertoire of strategies for finding out how people define their problems and their potential solutions within their particular circumstances.

1.18   A simple split between assessment and care management cannot be made: they should both be part of a continuous process.

The flexibility, sensitivity and variability of "care packages"

1.19   A package of care is not like a basket of goods and services; it is a fluid set of human relationships and arrangements. The care manager's main task will be to make the efforts of the people involved coherent; to ensure that the care of a dependent person is not dropped like the baton of a badly co-ordinated relay team. Teamwork is essential.

1.20   The machinery of contracting may make the response of service providers slower and too inflexible to meet the ever-changing nature of people's day to day relationships.

Local knowledge: the building blocks of "social" care planning

1.21   An unintended consequence of reforming children's services and community care at the same time is that many departments have set up separate planning processes and some are reorganising into children and adult divisions, rather than following the explicit recommendation of the proposals that "... the full range of social services authority functions should continue to form a coherent whole."

1.22   It is crucial that there should be "planning in the round" for all groups to ensure the development of coherent policy for the implementation of the Community Care and Children Acts reforms. In their efforts to ensure coherent policy and practice, some authorities have gone so far as to produce integrated "social care" plans. Such services should be built from the bottom up, based on the aggregate of local knowledge gained through partnerships with local people, assessments and the experience of negotiating packages of care.

Targeting services to those who need only a little intervention

1.23 A little help to many people in need is of enormous significance, be they individuals living at home or carers struggling to maintain others in the community. It is vital that resources are targeted on these people if the reforms are going to fulfil their aims.

Management implications in achieving effective collaboration

1.24 Where a degree of partnership with users, community groups, and other agencies at a local level has been achieved it has required a high degree of **participative management** to help the flow of planning information and devolution of decision making and resource allocation.

Specialist staff in locally-based teams and needs-led and community based services

1.25 Consultation with people in the community should be an integral part of, rather than follow reorganisation. Successful organisations are normally in a constant state of flux as they innovate to stay relevant to their changing circumstances.

1.26 A corollary of user-led services is a practice-led organisation. The place of specialist workers within the organisation will then vary according to the demands of the area.

1.27 The research supports small locally based generalist area **teams** and services, with specialists within them, rather than centralised services provided through specialist divisions based on administrative categories of "clients".

1.28 A matrix of geographically based and specialist worker teams needs to develop within the agency. A specialist division of labour requires good **teamwork** if coherence is to be established and maintained and the needs of the people are to be "managed" and not dropped as they pass from one person to another. Departments have to be able to demonstrate collaboration and teamwork of a high order **internally** as well as with other people and organisations in the community.

1.29   Mainstream social services tasks need to be handled through teamwork geared to the characteristics of special projects: relatively autonomous teams who have a detailed knowledge of the social situations they work with; the range of available resources located in local community groups, voluntary, not-for-profit or private agencies; the situations of the children and adults "in need" and those who care for them, and can be immediately responsive to changes in the lives of the people they work with.

1.30   Team development will be required with citizens and "professionals", at all levels within agencies and across organisational boundaries. Teamwork skills should be central to content and form of professional training and education.

Concluding notes: an expression of pessimism founded on optimism

1.31   Properly managed social services and social work departments, voluntary organisations and private agencies and good practice in the caring professions are a necessary but insufficient response to the challenges of community care. The right housing and income maintenance policies and adequate resources for social services are also crucial if people are to live independently.

1.32   A major fault in implementing the current reforms may prove to be a failure to build on people's normal capacity to care by overlooking the fact that carers and cared for can be given more support and choice by encouraging the involvement of a wider section of the community. There is a need to put in resources at times of crisis but these will not account for long-term care. This can only be provided by changes in patterns of care over time; by long-term development work, by directing professional time, expertise and energy at developing people's resources in the community; not just to target the "most needy" but also those social situations where care is most absent.

Chapter Two
Synthesis of the Research Findings

Introduction

2.1   The spirit of the legislation requires partnership between **all**
      those involved in community care for adults and child care,
      flexibility in devising packages of care, and a recognition that
      services need to be adaptable to local changes as well as to a
      wide variety of needs. The Seebohm report (para 474) referred to
      "a wider conception of social service, directed to the wellbeing of
      the whole of the community and not only of social casualties, and
      seeing the community it serves as the basis of its authority,
      resources and effectiveness". The report also spoke of dealing
      with people in response to their own definitions of need, in
      preference to the use of administrative or legal categorisations
      (Seebohm, 1968). These ideals have yet to be realised, and there
      are indications that administrative definitions continue to have
      the upper hand.

2.2   The new legislation provides another opportunity to improve the
      quality and accessibility of the personal social services. Yet the
      history of the Seebohm and the subsequent Barclay ideals warns
      against naive optimism. Success will require the political will to
      make available adequate resources at the right level of
      organisation; coherence between the policies of central
      government and local government, and a positive attitude toward
      developing the role and skills of social services and other staff in
      the statutory, independent and voluntary sectors. A balance needs
      to be achieved between targeting help to the most needy and
      delivering the small amounts of help at an early stage, crucial in
      preventing deterioration and crisis (Sinclair et al, 1990; Levin et
      al, 1989; Smale and Bennett, 1989; Darvill and Smale, 1990;
      Gibbons, 1990).

The process

2.3   The DoH guidelines for implementation of the new legislation
      were examined to identify a core group of common operational
      principles. These were in turn used in our trawl through the

literature to assist recognition of research findings which are relevant to the implementation process.

2.4 The operational principles adduced, which have been used as headings below, relate to:

- Collaboration between formal agencies.

- Collaboration with community groups/voluntary organisations representing user and carer interests.

- Planning as a product of negotiation between providers, users and carers.

- Assessment and care management.

- Combining value for money and monitoring quality of provision, having regard for users' choices.

Collaboration between formal agencies

2.5 The guidelines emphasise the importance of achieving collaboration between formal agencies, particularly in relation to policy objectives, joint planning, joint management, and developing a shared value base.

2.6 The importance of formal collaboration is detailed in the major publication *Working Together* (Consultation Paper Number 22 on the Children Act, 1989, DoH, June 1991). It is also called for in the Children Act: for example, the expectation on local authorities to co-ordinate the work of social services and education departments in the provision of day-care and pre-school activities:

"Co-operation between organisations, departments and individuals is crucial in the provision of protection for vulnerable children and also in ensuring proper use of available resources." (Department of Health, 1989 Chapter 2, para 41)

2.7 Studies show that effective collaboration between services is difficult to achieve (Sinclair et al, 1990) and necessitates:

- clarity about, and agreed separation of, their roles (Bayley et al, 1989);

- recognition that the achievement of shared values is not at odds with different approaches (Darvill and Smale, 1990 Chapter 6);

- managers and field staff learning about the roles of colleagues in other services (Bayley et al, 1989 p.165) as a prerequisite for collaboration in meeting the complexity of human needs;

- recognising that discussions between decision makers across agency boundaries are impeded by organisational resistance to change (Hadley et al, 1984 p.1) and by problems of split accountability to the organisation and to the inter-disciplinary collaborative machinery (Bayley et al, 1989 pp.167–8).

2.8   These issues require disciplined attention by managers and field staff alike and imply that, within each organisation, the relationship between managers and field staff needs to be reviewed. Not only do structures resist change (Hadley et al, 1984 p.1); the failure to integrate methods of working can be largely ascribed to managerial rigidity (Hadley and McGrath, 1984 p.10), and to the lack of consistent and shared ideology in management, in the professions, and in local teams (Hadley and McGrath, 1984 p.29).

2.9   Bayley et al (1989) showed that collaboration at a local level is most likely to take place when identification with the locality becomes more pressing than loyalty to the employing agency. Greater involvement with local people increases workers' accountability to them and can create tension between them and their organisational managers, to whom they are also accountable (Darvill and Smale, 1990). Black and minority ethnic group workers are often familiar with this conflict, both identifying with people in the community and being members of predominantly white organisations (Ahmad, 1990). Local level collaboration also requires convinced support by middle and senior management in order to avoid being constantly undermined (Crosbie and Vickery, 1989; Gibbons, 1990).

2.10   Effective team building with people from different agencies develops from three primary sources:

- increased understanding of each other's roles;

- the shared experience of working on a common task;

- the periodic acknowledgement of collective achievements. (Hadley and McGrath, 1984 p.140).

The nature of the collaboration should be negotiated through all levels of the organisation where staff and others are affected, to lead to effective outcomes. Gibbons demonstrated how collaboration over family and child care work between a social services department and three national voluntary child care organisations did not lead to meaningful partnerships at street level (Gibbons, 1990). There was little sharing in assessment and a low two-way flow of referrals.

2.11   Effective collaboration will require:

- investment in training for teamwork;

- setting realistic serial objectives (collaboration cannot be achieved by a single effort of will, but has to be worked at piecemeal);

- recognition that exclusive one-to-one working impedes collaboration;

- encouragement of innovation by managers, despite the risks and the administrative inconveniences involved in innovations (Hadley et al, 1987 pp.40, 137, 140; Smale and Tuson, 1990).

2.12   In short, collaboration **between** services depends in part on:

- the achievement of a sense of collaboration between the levels **within** each service;

- each service agreeing its aims and philosophy;

- management being participative;

- differences of perspective being resolved;

- there being flexibility in organisational roles;

- attitudes towards contingent services becoming positive;

- recognition that internal integration takes time (Hadley et al, 1987 pp.120–1, 133, 152).

2.13   For collaboration to permeate the whole organisation through to the "street-level" there has to be more effective teamwork, a move away from individualised perceptions of the problem, and individualised ways of organising work.

2.14   Studies of care management schemes conducted by the Personal Social Services Research Unit in Kent and Gateshead (Challis and Davies, 1986; Challis et al, 1990) underline the importance of teamwork and team-building and the need for organisations to develop new team structures which address new perceptions of the problems they are set up to tackle. Characteristic processes involve the necessity of creating a "team ethos" across different disciplinary groupings by locating all members in the same office.

2.15   Their research underlines the significance of facilitating change and sometimes creating "teams" or "care networks", specific to each user, including the service user, formal and informal carers and a range of professionals. The need to recognise that "a package of care" is in practice "a team of people" is discussed in Chapter Three. It is a more extended idea of "teamwork", but one which is supported by the Kent and Gateshead experience. **A team is that group of people who depend on each other to some extent to complete the task.** There are many factors involved in this extended view of teamwork which are alluded to in the PSSRU research but which are not explicitly described and analysed.

2.16   Teamwork, between staff from different agencies, within the agency, and between professionals and citizens, is crucial. Smale and Tuson (1989), working with innovatory practitioners from different agencies, found that this need for teamwork in practice necessitates a review of the base of social work education, training and continuing staff development.

Collaboration and elderly people

2.17   Sinclair et al (1990) in their review of research on welfare provision for elderly people suggest that a policy which aims to secure an adequate standard of care that is reliable and which reaches the most disabled elderly people throughout the UK must be built around a strong statutory sector. The voluntary and private sectors will have an important role, especially where they have traditionally been strong, and in services which they have traditionally provided. However "an overemphasis on private and voluntary sectors may lead to a loss of their presumed virtues, turning both sectors into expensively monitored means of providing state-funded services which are not innovatory, challenging or consumer-led, nor distributed according to need" (Sinclair et al, 1990 p.387).

2.18   They emphasise the interdependence of the services that enable people to live an abundant life, such as housing, heating and transport. Financial savings cannot be made by targeting or repackaging care, but only by reducing the amount and the standard of care ". . . and that in a moral sense is no care at all."

Admirable policies are already in place, but provision is patchy. Unless resources are considerably increased reforms will merely benefit one group of old people at the expense of another. Differences between areas in their affluence and private/voluntary resources should be acknowledged. Excessive confidence as to how the three sectors might work together could result in a weak statutory sector which is unable to respond to the omissions of the others (Sinclair et al, 1990). A useful method of assessing the strengths of an area's networks has been triggered by Tennant and Bayley(1985).

2.19   These authorities pointed out that collaboration in community care requires effective coordination of central government policies, good relationships between central and local government and effective communication between their agents, such as health authorities, housing departments, social services departments and social security offices. Poor coordination of services within social service departments has been demonstrated. More will be expected of the complex and diverse private and voluntary services; and we enter a period of fundamental change for the NHS.

2.20   Sinclair and his colleagues argue that there is not an efficient market mechanism because there is no generally agreed medium of exchange, and information as to what can be provided on what grounds is lacking. There are monopoly suppliers and a curious assortment of provisions governed by entitlements and cash limits. Availability restricts the choice of consumers: in practice a frail elderly person supported by social security and her relatives may be allocated to a private home as providing the only vacancy in her area.

2.21   Rational planning is also problematic. There is a lack of agreed criteria as to what the system should be: planners do not have the information required for planning, nor can they compel those outside their organisation to do what is required of them. Planners come from different professions, confront different planning cycles and geographical areas and have different objectives.

2.22   Collaboration may be feasible for specific issues but it may prove impossible to involve all agencies and sectors in some grand overall design, even at the local level. Hence the need for a strong statutory sector to identify and plug the gaps left by others (pp. 382-3). Moreover "collaboration is no substitute for resources.

At present an adequate and coordinated package of services for one person must mean that no services are available at all for others who might need them" (Sinclair et al, 1990).

Collaboration with community groups/voluntary organisations representing user and carer interests

2.23 Collaboration with community groups and others is emphasised in the community care reforms. This emphasis is grounded in a preference for informal over formal modes of care, a recognition of the importance of the social context of user needs, and identification of the necessity for professional staff to foster collaboration with informal carers.

2.24 These same three aspects of collaboration are evident in the Children Act and its underlying principles. **Firstly**, there is clearly a preference for "informal" care in the sense of:

● care provided by the child's family;

● the need for developing and maintaining a working partnership with parents;

● the maintenance of family links if "formal" care is necessary.

Collaboration at this level will also be necessary for local authorities to carry out their new duty "to promote the upbringing of children in need by their families so far as is consistent with their welfare".

Secondly, the Act recognises the importance of the social context of children, and children in need:

"Although some basic needs are universal, there can be a variety of ways of meeting them. Patterns of family life differ according to culture, class and community and these differences should be respected and accepted. There is no one, perfect way to bring up children and care must be taken to avoid value judgements and stereotyping." (Chapter 2, para 2)

Thirdly, the Children Act demands collaboration with parents and other care-givers. For example, "... measures which antagonise, undermine, or marginalise parents are counter-productive" (para.1) and "... parents should be expected and enabled to retain their responsibilities ..." (para 12).

2.25   There is no discrete division between these aspects of
        collaboration and the issue about formal organisations working
        together, as illustrated by the following passages concerning
        social work with children and families and with elderly people
        living alone, and the voluntary sector.

2.26   These issues can be addressed through a single question: how can
        formal agencies change to work better alongside the community?
        Gibbons (1990) concluded that it would be easier to implement
        policies which call for a switch of emphasis to locally-based,
        independent provision if agencies allowed time and gave
        recognition to the development work of managers on the one hand
        and freed workers from caseloads on the other hand. Workers in
        the second category might not be professional social workers.
        Crosbie and Vickery (1989) also found that collaboration between
        staff and voluntary groups was much more likely to last where
        managers supported initiatives carried out by staff with specific
        skills within a geographically based generalist team. (The role
        of specialism within locally-based teams is discussed in Chapter
        Three.)

2.27   Sommerlad and Webb (1988) confirmed the value of small units
        geared to provide a range of support specifically to self-help
        groups, i.e. self-help support projects such as the eighteen funded
        by the Self-Help Alliance. They concluded:

        "The single most important rationale for a (self-help support
        project's) role in improving access is the inability of statutory
        agencies to communicate effectively to users of its services. The
        project:

        ●   does basic intelligence work;

        ●   it clarifies roles and responsibilities;

        ●   it identifies useful and sympathetic professionals; and,

        ●   it sets up direct links that can be used by people in need."

2.28   A study by Van der Eyken of Homestart's voluntary visiting
        schemes for at-risk families demonstrated the value of these
        schemes to the families. The families themselves, the volunteers
        and professionals in touch with the families all rated as high
        the level of change in family behaviour which volunteers could
        facilitate. The independence of the volunteers was felt to be
        important (Van der Eyken, 1982).

Social work and elderly people living alone

2.29 The London borough studied by the Networks project (Sinclair et al, 1988) was found to be well-provided with both statutory and voluntary services and was therefore not necessarily typical or average. The area team services, especially the home help service, had achieved an impressive degree of coverage of certain elderly groups, suggesting that social workers looking for partners in the community could well begin by looking to their own colleagues in the home-help service. There was a strong case for co-ordination and collaboration between the three area services (occupational therapy, home help and social work) based on:

- coverage: 85% of the elderly people in touch with the area office in any one week being in touch with the home help service;

- overlap: home-helps attending half the occupational therapy clients, nearly two-thirds of the social work allocated elderly clients and more than four in ten of elderly referrals to those services;

- client similarity in social characteristics;

- relationship with neighbours: the home help service being the only one with sufficient local presence to be aware of day-to-day changes in the provision of neighbourly help.

2.30 Close collaboration between the social services department's own services should bring benefits to collaboration with people in the community . Social workers and occupational therapists could get early warning from home helps on any deterioration in the client's use of aids. Social work innovations such as the development of self-help groups could become more accessible to home-help clients. Home-helps should have access to advice on how to manage their more "difficult" clients, such as those who were confused.

2.31 However, co-ordination within the department was hampered in several respects. At the level of work with individuals there were no formal procedures whereby one service informed another about a case. Time spent by home helps in discussing particular cases immediately resulted in a direct loss in time available to spend with clients. Because of the numbers of home helps social workers rarely shared more than one case with a particular home help so that the benefits of a good working relationship established in one case could not easily be transferred to others.

Moreover, budgeting constraints, different traditions of management in the home help and social work services, central control over staffing and unclear or conflicting priorities all contributed to making flexible coordination difficult. The development of "care management" systems will hopefully bring the coordination necessary to overcome some of these problems. But it should be noted that whereas a "care manager" may be well placed to coordinate services from "providers" within the department or from the independent sector, the home helps are in a pivotal position for the coordination of the "informal" aspect of "care packages" with paid-for services.

2.32   The workload management systems identified by the research were appropriate for accounting for work with individuals rather than organising for common action based on neighbourhood or shared difficulties (Sinclair et al, 1988 p.85). Evidence from the Schemes project (Crosbie and Vickery, 1989) and from family support (Gibbons, 1990) and community based development work (Darvill and Smale, 1990) have all stressed the need for "workload management" systems that give proper place to interagency collaboration and community development activities, as opposed to narrow "caseload" management systems focusing only on individualised work.

2.33   It may be noted that the services discussed are in fact parts of a "whole" social services department and that collaboration with people in the community rested on partnerships, or teamwork within the agency. We consider that the views quoted about a need for collaboration support the view that these provisions should be combined into one service at geographical area level, with a specialist division of labour within the area team. (See Chapter Three.)

The voluntary sector, unpaid neighbours and the development of local resources

2.34   The voluntary sector encompasses self-help and neighbourhood groups as well as major voluntary organisations and voluntary helpers. The statutory sector needs to put a new emphasis on the social infrastructure, seeing and acknowledging the resources that exist.

2.35   The agenda for discussion of care of the elderly has been radically altered in the last 15–20 years (Sinclair et al, 1990). Emphasis has moved from institutional care to care in the community, and from the statutory sector to a mixed pattern of provision by statutory, voluntary, informal and, increasingly, the commercial sectors. Sinclair and his colleagues point out that many now consider the welfare state to be in crisis, due to disenchantment with the services provided. Statutory provision may cost too much and through its bureaucracy lead to inefficient and unresponsive services, while the informal and voluntary sectors are commonly assumed to be cheaper, more responsive to needs, flexible, providing better quality care and encouraging responsibility and discouraging dependence. Many of these assumptions are unproven and much theorising about the role of the voluntary sector is based on potential strengths rather than historical and current realities. The emphasis on service delivery could lead to a distortion of the voluntary sector; taking them away from campaigning, advocacy and innovation, a process already causing concern in the Black community (Jones, 1991).

2.36   Studies reviewed by Sinclair et al suggested that:

- voluntary organisations are more numerous in middle-class areas and that where there is already a relatively active voluntary sector, more new voluntary projects are generated (Hatch and Mocroft, 1970; Leat et al, 1986);

- availability of volunteers is unevenly spread between groups (Hatch, 1978);

- neighbourhood care groups are more active in some areas than others (Abrams et al, 1981);

- local authorities may be generous with funds and yet have few specific arrangements for encouraging voluntary-statutory co-operation in planning and co-ordinating new services (Moore and Green, 1985; Leat et al, 1986);

- social workers' attitudes are important for the involvement of volunteers and voluntary organisations (Hatch et al, 1981; Holme and Maizels, 1978);

- where local authority social services were most decentralised and/or where specialist posts had been created, social workers were more likely to work with voluntary groups (Hatch et al, 1981);

- who receives services may be related to prevailing ideas about responsibilities for care, i.e. male carers may be more likely than females to seek and receive services (Parker, 1985);

- volunteers' perceptions of need play an important part in determining the practical criteria for allocation (Abrams, 1978; Leat, 1979; Hadley et al, 1975);

- professionals may be unwilling to refer clients to voluntary projects, especially in the early stages (Abrams et al, 1981; Moore and Green, 1985; Leat, 1983);

- due to misperceptions about what volunteers can do, social workers may either fail to refer dependent clients or refer them inappropriately (Power, 1979; Levin et al, 1983);

- once a professional has used a scheme he or she is likely to use it again (Moore and Green, 1985; Leat, 1983);

- carers may prefer to pay for services because this reduces a sense of indebtedness and hence allows them to use the service more often (Moore and Green, 1985).

2.37   Studies regarding the effectiveness of the voluntary sector suggest that the effectiveness of voluntary visiting might be improved if the allocation procedures were improved and more attention paid to matching volunteers and clients (Hadley et al, 1975; Shenfield and Allen, 1972). Day care for elderly people has a variable impact on their physical and mental health (Edwards and Carter, 1980; MacDonald et al, 1982), and one of its main functions may be to relieve carers (Brocklehurst and Tucker, 1980). The presence of a paid organiser is desirable for success (Chisholm and Fletcher, 1979; Mendel, 1979 a,b). Voluntary carer-support services have been underfunded and underused and subject to vagaries of funding (Moore and Green, 1985). There is a lack of knowledge concerning consumer preferences, such as under what conditions volunteer support is acceptable. Moreover, a study of a range of innovatory schemes designed to help people at home concluded that good neighbour, warden and alarm schemes should be seen as part of a package of care tailored to individual needs (Tinker, 1984).

2.38   In sum, the voluntary sector is haphazard in geography, funding, activities and relationships with local statutory policies and personnel.

2.39   Five suggestions are offered as to how to retain the strengths of the voluntary sector while recognising the needs of the statutory sector to ensure equity and accountability:

- payment of volunteers may increase the supply and render volunteers more acceptable to social workers, through a contract or means of control;

- purchase of service contracting may overcome some of the weaknesses of the voluntary sector although it cannot overcome existing unequal distribution of voluntary services;

- a re-orientation of social work education could change attitudes of professionals so that referrals make the best use of the services;

- planning and management skills need to be developed and mechanisms devised for adequate co-ordination both within and between voluntary and statutory bodies;

- an information campaign might bring forth more volunteers and inform people about services available (Sinclair et al, 1990).

2.40 The work described by the innovative practitioners involved in the Community Social Work Exchange (Smale and Bennett, 1989; Darvill and Smale, 1990) and that researched by Hadley and McGrath (1984) and Bayley and his colleagues (1989) gives a different perception of the relationship between "professional" and "voluntary" support. These locally based teams and projects have demonstrated that it is possible to develop relationships with a wide range of people in the community and break down the normal barriers between "professionals" and "volunteers" within an active strategy of partnership. This increases the range and variety of responses available to local people to choose from when they require help with a wide range of problems across "client" groups. These ways of working also enable a broad spectrum of people, some of whom would be seen as "clients" in more orthodox settings, to engage in "service provision", thus breaking down the divisions between "providers" and "users", a distinction which is probably only relevant when a cash transaction is the route to care.

Black voluntary organisations

2.41 Bandana Ahmad identifies Black voluntary organisations as a resource for change. In the past they have fared badly in the competition for resources and status. Among the characteristics of Black agencies are that they:

- provide alternative services;

- deal with all aspects of a community's needs or, when dealing with a particular need such as mental health, take a comprehensive approach;

- have little or no regional boundaries;

- have access to severely restricted resources and hence suffer greater insecurity than most mainstream voluntary organisations;

- offer relatively poor training opportunities and terms and conditions for staff.

2.42 She thinks that some "white" or "mainstream" voluntary agencies have acted with determination to improve their services to Black people and a noticeable change in the attitudes and perceptions of social services departments is commented on. Social workers can contribute to the process of change by:

- informing themselves about local and national Black voluntary organisations;

- acting as a personal resource;

- making reference to Black organisations as a matter of routine practice, instead of normally making reference to white organisations;

- checking how prepared white organisations are in meeting the racial and cultural needs of their Black client(s), when references to white organisations are made;

- using the expertise of Black voluntary organisations not just to empower Black clients, but also to avoid exploiting them as "dumping grounds";

- learning from these organisations about how to work within the framework of a "holistic" approach and incorporate this approach in social work assessment and intervention;

- forming partnerships with Black organisations in gaining resources and support from their own and other agencies;

- establishing a trusting relationship with Black organisations (Ahmad, B, 1990).

2.43 Jones has pointed out that the purchasing and contracting aspects of the new legislation have considerable implications for Black voluntary organisations. Many local authorities have rapidly completed deals with large "white" voluntary organisations which "too often have appalling records of institutional racism".

Evidence of local community participation is recommended as a way of ensuring that future contractors do not perpetuate this problem. Some local authorities will now only consider funding voluntary groups who can contract for specific community care services, leading to groups being rushed into providing services while lacking structures and resources for co-ordination and development of services, negotiating and preparing contracts, and quality control. Contracting to provide services excludes other community groups from the campaigning activities for which they were set up, shifting them from their original aims (Jones, 1991).

A political preference for informal over formal modes of care

2.44   In moving towards greater relative use of informal and voluntary groupings, certain general issues will need to be addressed:

- It is naive to assume that local supportive networks exist "in nature" (Bulmer, 1986; Hadley et al, 1987 p.97; Smale et al, 1988); all studies show that to develop networks and to improve informal community resources requires the appointment and development of workers with motivation and skills (Sinclair et al, 1988; Bayley, 1989; Crosbie and Vickery, 1989; Smale and Tuson, 1988). It is necessary to emphasise the importance of managerial responsibility for this kind of appointment and for harnessing the knowledge of networks (their maintenance and development) to the tasks of care managers and service providers. There is the risk that crisis work will prevent essential developmental work, and the dependence on the voluntary sector will not be accompanied by a sense of responsibility and accountability towards it.

- Recent trends towards specialised divisions based on client groupings may be moving workers and service co-ordination and provision away from a base in neighbourhoods and from a comprehensive understanding of the social context of people's lives.

- There can sometimes be a conflict in practice between emphasis on targeting help to the most needy and the epidemiological approach to needs which the legislation requires through community care planning and surveying the needs of children in the area. Targeting should not deny all professional help to needy people who are not in a targeted group. The longer term consequences of such exclusions should be charted.

- Most clients prefer highly personal forms of care to be undertaken by paid workers when relatives are not available, rather than by volunteers, in contrast to befriending functions which can be undertaken by neighbours (Sinclair et al, 1988; 1990).

- Recent government attitudes have been perceived by many as removing power from local authories and disempowering professional workers. It may be unrealistic to expect those authorities and workers to exercise the imagination and innovation required by the legislation, and to engage in processes of local empowerment. Community-based collaborative schemes will require pump-priming, though no additional funding is anticipated, except for mental health, if they are not to exploit volunteers and carers (Hadley et al, 1984 pp.15, 253).

2.45   The kinds of local collaboration envisaged in the guidelines constitute one of the most difficult aspects of future change. The following indicates the contribution of action-research to this process.

2.46   Innovations in practice tend to be generated by a small team of enthusiasts, working on issues with local appeal, and feeling a sense of ownership for their work. The written word, including directives from above, are insufficient to change practice (Crosbie et al, 1989 pp.15–16). Mutual enthusiasm and teamwork with local people depend on shared commitment to information-gathering and service planning, periodic evaluation, genuine participation and a sense of partnership with local people, the development of contracts, and effective management of the workloads of both paid staff and volunteers (Smale and Bennet, 1989 pp.21, 39–40, 61–63). Where the statutory services employ specialist workers, it is essential that they should not be seen as divorced from the local community: i.e. collaboration is not possible between "insiders" and "outsiders" (Crosbie et al, 1989 p. 181). Similarly, those engaged solely in individual or family casework must be seen to be associated in some way with community development activities (Smale et al, 1988; Darvill and Smale, 1990 pp.14–15).

2.47   Abrams challenged easy assumptions about the complementarity of formal and informal care. The idea of a complementary "interweaving" of the formal and the informal is challenged by the possibility of conflictful and other modes of relationship. He describes the strategic ways in which the formal and the informal sectors relate to each other, and illustrates these from the research studies. Organisations involved in developing partnership with the informal sector will need to recognise the possibilities for colonization, conflict, coexistence and confusion. They will need to be explicit about what kinds of relationships they need, and be able to analyse unforeseen consequences of their activities which unwittingly draw them into undesired types of relationships with the informal sector (Bulmer, 1986).

2.48   Effective statutory-voluntary collaboration in service provision depends on:

- the location of the work within organisational and community structures;

- the workers' sense of accountability to the local community;

- partnership with local people (for examples see Darvill and Smale, 1990 p.103 et seq.; Smale and Bennett, 1989).

Statutory workers need to know about and to appreciate informal care, and to be skilled in supporting the complex forms which local caring may take (Bayley et al, 1989 pp.2, 103, 163). The systems approach to social work is useful in these respects (Bayley et al, 1989 p.13 Part II; Smale et al, 1988), not least because this addresses:

- the issues in professionalism raised by local involvement;

- relationships with non-professionals;

- appropriate delegation (Bayley et al, 1989 pp.172–3).

There are major skills involved in achieving **both** partnerships with residents in which there is **mutual** learning, issues of power differentials that have to be recognised and addressed **and** the maintenance of professional integrity and authority (Darvill and Smale, 1990 Chapters 3,4 and 6).

Recognition of the importance of the social context of clients' perception of their needs

2.49   "Modern neighbourhoodism is in its purest form an attempt by newcomers to create a local social world through political or quasi-political action. Great organisational skills and ingenious organisational devices are often used in attempts to mobilise old and new residents alike in order to protect amenities, enhance resources and, to a greater or lesser degree, wrench control of the local milieu from outside authorities and vest it in strictly local hands." (Bulmer, 1986 p.95)

2.50   This vision of a modern neighbourhoodism, grounded in the research into neighbourhood care schemes, carries significant implications for community care. It implies that modern social conditions do have this creative potential which professional agencies will need to be explicitly working with—or against, at the local level. Its politicised nature, "the political voice of local attachment", will be particularly significant the more professional agencies devolve, decentralise, listen to the user and so forth. Understanding and being able to work with these localised political movements will be increasingly crucial. Attention has also been drawn to the need to address the poverty of the context, as well as problems of the individual (Gibbons, 1990).

Localisation

2.51   A conclusion from Abrams' studies of neighbourhoods and neighbourhood care schemes is the heterogeneity of both. People's background culture and position in society will inevitably cause them to see their social problems differently, just as it will affect their perception of community neighbourhood and what is normal in the community.

2.52   Sufficiently sensitive understanding of the nature of neighbouring and the way neighbour relationships mesh or otherwise with other social relationships in a particular area, particularly friendships and kinships, will require detailed local knowledge. Such knowledge can only be obtained by equally heterogeneous methods adapted to the character of particular localities and particular social networks (Bulmer, 1986; Hearn and Thompson, 1987; Smale et al, 1988; Smale and Tuson, 1988).

Subjectivity

2.53   Abrams wrote that neighbourhoods and neighbouring are as much subjective perceptions as objective facts: ". . . territorial bounding is determined subjectively, not by administrative maps and plans . . . My effective neighbourhood may be quite different from that of my next-door neighbour" (Bulmer, 1986 p.238). An understanding

of such subjectivities becomes crucial (
Perspectives Exchange, 1990).

Social class

2.54 "We are impelled to the vi
most important sources of vari..
in which people actually succeed o..
neighbourly environment they desire. Bu..
to the view that in one form or another neighb..
deeply cherished, strenuously pursued value of all s..
classes and groups and one which social policy ought to be
more constructively seeking to realise". (Bulmer, 1986 p.12)

2.55 Understanding the kinds of informal care actually occurring in
particular social networks, and understanding what the potential
for change in such networks might be, involves understanding the
particular social class composition of the members of those
networks. For example, "Under certain circumstances, working
class people evidently do participate substantially in
neighbourhood care" (Bulmer, 1986 p.161). Understanding what
these "certain circumstances" are would be essential for
understanding this particular dimension of informal care. Again
Abrams provides descriptive analysis of the social class
dimension in several specific and concrete examples which
underline the general point.

2.56 The effectiveness and responsiveness of community social work
experiments have frequently depended on a community-oriented
and participative style of management (Hadley and McGrath,
1984 pp.257–8; Smale et al, 1988 Chapter 6), and on managerial
recognition—despite the individualistic stance of all welfare
legislation—that the client-centred approach tends to ignore
local networks (Hadley and McGrath, 1984 p.8). Where problems
have arisen in developing responsive local services, these are
frequently associated with organisational/ managerial conflicts
concerning local management versus centralised priorities, lateral
versus vertical forms of accountability, and the nature and content
of work-evaluation (Crosbie et al, 1989 pp.83, 86). Practical
guidance is available in Darvill and Smale (1990 pp.32, 35–6,
49–50, 54–6) on the conduct of local network conferences,
developing a typology of local networks, developing caring
networks, and promoting teamwork. Further guidance may be
found in Smale et al (1988) on reviewing decision making within

.ents, recognising the reciprocity of relationships and
ρing structures which do not inhibit innovation.

e need for workers in the statutory sector to develop
ctitudes which foster collaboration with informal helpers

Attitudinal change is interdependent with organisational,
managerial and professional changes (Bayley et al, 1989 p.51).
Attitudes which need to be fostered in seeking collaboration with
local helpers and resources are commitment to:

- an interlocking system of teams;

- flexibility of tasks;

- informality of approach (Bayley et al, 1989 p.163; Smale
  et al, 1988 Chapter 3);

- becoming part of the informal networks (Hadley et al, 1987
  pp.101–5; Smale et al, 1988 Chapter 6). (See below).

2.58   The professional task of social workers needs to be based upon
        determination to maintain flexible responses at field level, and
        commitment to responsive experimentation in localities. The
        constants are:

- the search for partnership with clients, co-workers and other
  helpers;

- enhancing a sense of openness and choice;

- ensuring that effective work should also be efficient in
  resource terms;

- blurring the divisions between management and practice since
  both should be proactive in planning local services.

Reviews are required of:

- systems of communication and supervision within agencies;

- collective definitions of accountability;

- the practice of linking organisational roles exclusively to
  specific levels of employment (Sainsbury, 1990).

2.59   Issues relevant to these headings, although they may not be
        helpfully associated with specific guidelines, are to be found in
        NISW's Schemes research project.

Schemes

2.60 Crosbie and Vickery's examination of schemes for old people in six areas differentiates between those which were controlled entirely by social services and those set up in partnership with community groups and organisations.

2.61 Partnerships are classified according to whether they are involved with:

- community groups;

- "secondary volunteers" whose primary attachment was to another enterprise, e.g. school or church;

- established voluntary organisations, e.g. Age Concern;

- newly formed voluntary organisations established specifically to run the scheme.

2.62 The amount of staff time needed for each type of partnership depended on the social infrastructure of the area, the scale of the scheme, and the degree to which the volunteers already had organisational skills.

2.63 In most of the schemes, particularly those run by secondary volunteers and established voluntary organisations, the area office provided a "springboard" (Adams, 1986). This required high initial input of staff time but later led to virtual independence of the scheme from direct involvement of area staff. In a few areas the setting up of schemes was dependent on the adoption by the area offices of a community development strategy requiring long term involvement with community groups.

2.64 Where new voluntary organisations with paid staff were seen to be required social services could be heavily involved and the process of designing the scheme and obtaining finance for it could be prolonged.

2.65 Additional practical reasons for area staff involvement were to co-ordinate the needs of two client groups, as when one group was providing services for another (e.g. young offenders on an intermediate treatment programme undertaking gardening for older people); and when special skills or knowledge of working with elderly persons were required, but were lacking in the intended "partner organisation".

2.66   The research contrasted two main strategies that an area office might adopt towards promoting schemes: retaining social services department control and setting up partnerships. The advantage of retaining control was that schemes could be located and targeted according to the judgment of the social services department rather than decisions of outside bodies. They could be integrated with existing services to make use of social services' expertise. However, such schemes were vulnerable to unplanned closure due to competing demands on staff time or even poor collaboration within the department. Moreover, the tying up of finite resources on a long term basis meant staff were less liable to develop new schemes. (A manual concerning implementation of schemes has recently been produced by Miller et al, 1991.)

Partnerships in schemes

2.67   Partnership schemes could be handed over to external people and therefore required less staff time and commitment (Crosbie and Vickery, 1989). But in order to develop community resources in deprived areas staff needed to engage in long-term community development activities, such as support of community groups. Achieving local community involvement in partnerships with voluntary organisations was difficult, although these organisations might be better able to achieve a wide coverage of need or save resources for the social services (Crosbie and Vickery, 1989 pp.104–5).

2.68   Partnerships proved appropriate for developing clubs and support schemes for elderly and disabled people, and play groups. Partnerships were not so frequent in schemes close to the statutory aspects of social work, such as schemes for difficult adolescents, foster parents or childminders.

2.69   The researchers pointed out a potential conflict between providing an imaginative programme needing particular skills to implement it and the wish to involve outsiders. Handing over control too hastily could result in a loss of focus and purpose, such as reminiscence work being replaced by bingo. It was important to recognise where special skills were required and should be retained (Crosbie and Vickery, 1989 pp.93–4).

2.70   In another study of professional intervention and helping networks informal care provided to elderly people living at home was found to be inhibited by:

●   clients' attitudes of reluctance to accept practical help from informal supporters, especially neighbours;

- carer specialization, such as emergency surveillance given only by neighbours, and intimate confiding restricted to children;

- carer variability, or differences in what carers could offer.

2.71   The absence of children or their inability or unwillingness to provide care in particular cases was an important limitation on informal care (Sinclair et al, 1988 pp.49, 66).

Self-help groups: support workers and professionals

2.72   Professional workers have a crucial but very delicate role in supporting self-help groups. Vincent (1986) showed how groups are more likely to be run on participative rather than authoritarian lines, and to be longer-lasting, where professionals offered support. Groups which can progress without support may consist of those already best able to help themselves. Richardson (1983) demonstrated how the self-help groups most vulnerable to collapse were those which attracted people for short crisis periods rather than for on-going help, and where the main need was for practical help rather than social support. Single-parent self-help groups were particularly vulnerable to disintegration on that basis.

2.73   Abraham and Webb (1989), as part of the Tavistock Institute evaluation of the Self-Help Alliance, identified that professionals need to be sensitive to the different value-bases of self-help groups in the mental health field. These include: anti-medical; alternative therapy; anti-psychiatry; women's movement; race and ethnicity; community development; "pre self-help". The research showed how these groups benefit from operating as part of a mix of: worker-led time-limited groups; worker-led drop ins; self-run groups; and a telephone network.

Participation and constraints on informal care

2.74   Very small sums of financial support can also have a strong symbolic significance over and above their monetary value (Richardson, 1983). Gibbons showed how family centres which are available to a whole population, not only to those in greatest need, can contribute to greater participation in wider community issues. About a fifth of those in contact with centres took on responsibility and acquired a range of relevant new skills (Gibbons, 1990).

Religion

2.75 When looking at the characteristics of helpers in organised neighbourhood care, Abrams found that the role of religion was very important, especially as only two out of the ten projects studied had any overt religious connections. He recognised that this might be interpreted in many ways, for example, as evidence of "the life cycle organisation of religiosity" (Bulmer, 1986 p.161), but nevertheless concluded that "however unselfconsciously, . . . background ideologies identifying altruism as a moral absolute are one important factor explaining participation in neighbourhood care of an organised sort". The significance of religious beliefs in the development of support in Black and ethnic minority groups has also been stressed (Ahmad, B, 1990).

2.76 The activities of religious organisations as a centre of help and care is a dimension of local social relationships which staff of welfare agencies need to be aware of, and need to be able to relate to effectively (Bulmer, 1986).

Family and kinship

2.77 "Something like nine-tenths of the care given to those who in various ways cannot fend for themselves in our society is given by spouses, parents, children and other kin . . . The ideal of domiciliary care proclaimed by the vast majority of those actually and prospectively in need of care is in effect a blunt preference for the family." (Bulmer, 1986 p.233)

2.78 Abrams saw this fact as the heart of informal care. Care by kin is founded on reciprocity and competence, hence the task of improving care requires "a deepening and re-inforcing" of commitment; the "building of functional equivalents among non-kin"; the development of competence of carers; and the enhancement of reciprocity. The type of tasks undertaken by different relatives will vary with cultural differences. There are also differences in the tasks typically performed by men and women. The development of "self-help" organisations is seen as a good example of the creation of a context for reciprocity.

2.79 Child care studies have shown that statutory workers pay insufficient regard to intra-family links, changes in family structures, and the value which parents place on being consulted by the professionals (DoH, 1985 pp.10, 12). It has been noted that professional assessments are weakest in the exploration of kinship and neighbourhood networks (Rowe, 1985 p.13; Packman, 1986), in their dependence on implicit unproven assumptions about need and disposal, and dependence on professional ideology at the expense of local knowledge (Rowe, 1985 p.17). Rowe suggests that these defects are not simply professional failure, but result indirectly from the unresponsiveness of large bureaucracies; this implies, therefore, that managers should give special attention to enhancing their workers' knowledge of kinship and local networks, and how to preserve these networks (Rowe, 1985 pp.20, 43).

2.80   It is not easy, because of bureaucratic structures and the professional emphasis on clients' inadequacies rather than strengths, to listen to the voice of service-users and those who represent them, or to share control with them in determining policies and provisions (Bayley, 1989 pp.6, 168, 171). These difficulties are compounded by gender, class and ethnic minority differences between workers and clients and the diversity, or absences , of professional practice models, many of which concentrate on individual psychological functioning at the expense of awareness of the social situation (Smale et al, 1991). Yet health and welfare are not simply technical matters for the disposal of experts: see Bayley on "interweaving" and the integration of services (pp.3, 164, 171). Time needs to be made available, therefore, for statutory workers to identify the extent and characteristics of neighbourhoods and networks (Hadley et al, 1987 pp.57–8), and for their managers to develop the following specific skills: leadership, interpersonal skills in **open** discussions, political and entrepreneurial sophistication, achieving clarity concerning the limits of delegation, striking balances between local autonomy and service-accountability, and community involvement (Hadley et al, 1987 pp.201–3, 209, 217; Challis et al, 1990 p.9).

2.81   These findings about the importance of family and kinship ties, and the weakness of professional understanding of the necessity for maintaining them, is reinforced by more recent studies. For example:

> "Evidence from a number of studies shows that no matter if family links have been weak, or turbulent, most children and young people who experience care do return to their parents or at least to some member of their family ..." (DoH, 1990b p. 22)

2.82   In a discussion of the Dartington Research Unit's study of children in care, and the follow-up study of access disputes about children in care, the authors conclude:

"If children remain in care for two years or more away from home, four-fifths of them will experience severe barriers to maintaining contact with their parents ... As a result, a third of those who remain in care will have lost contact with mother or father, siblings or the wider family at the end of two years and will be likely to stay in care for the foreseeable future. In the majority of cases, there are no cogent social work reasons for contact with the family to wither ....". (DoH, 1990b p.26)

Black people and ethnic minorities

2.83   It has been demonstrated that black and minority ethnic elders generally do experience "triple jeopardy" (Norman, 1985): suffer the effects of racism; are disadvantaged in housing, health, employment and pensions; and services are not tailored to their general and specific needs. Variety in provision is required and should arise from genuine links between statutory, voluntary agencies, user representatives and local people rather than tokenistic gestures made for short term political ends.

2.84   Abrams' work did not separately identify race as a significant variable in either the street studies or the neighbourhood care schemes. The main conclusion was:

"One substantive aspect of neighbouring and neighbourhood care which requires more attention is the relationship between residential proximity and inter-ethnic co-operation and conflict. Tattworth was a racially mixed area, but the research as a whole may give the impression that whereas class, age, sex, and religious affiliation are sociologically significant criteria, race or ethnicity are not. Clearly, if this impression is given it would be misleading, and more research is needed". (Bulmer, 1986 p.237)

2.85   Jenny Williams writes in *The Kaleidoscope of Care* research review on the difficulty of commenting on services for elders from Black and minority ethnic communities because of the shortcomings of existing literature. Some topics, such as the health needs of Black and ethnic minority elders, have not yet been fully addressed and "the mainstream tradition of empirical and largely quantitative analysis sits uneasily beside the historical and qualitative approach of some of the literature on these elders. The quantitative approach may indeed be an inappropriate tool to explore the complex conceptual and emotional aspects of life for old people in Black and ethnic minority groups" (Sinclair et al, 1990).

2.86   She suggests that such enquiries as have used quantitative methods have often lacked the methodological rigour necessary for statistical comparability and generalisation usually considered necessary for planned changes in policy and practice. For example, there has been little systematic comparison with white elderly control groups matched for age and social class. Since the research reviewed has largely focused on local and specific groups it lacks generalisation to other areas where elders have different ethnic origins or have experienced different life conditions.

2.87   Dutt and Ahmad (1991) argue for a different view of research. They suggest that premises informing the methodology of research about Black people have been too often based in an ideology that perceives Black people as victims and reinforces stereotypes. Hence the methodology does not benefit either Black people as individuals, or the community; self-determination of Black people is inhibited and access to services is obstructed. They propose a Black perspective, which will reinforce people's strengths, while acknowledging requirements and duties. The methodology should benefit individuals and the Black community generally, resulting in mechanisms to raise awareness within the Black community and organisations providing services. The relationship of researcher and subject should be of mutual benefit, and a process of partnership. An example offered is of an examination of the needs of Black elders in which individuals' assessments were translated into offers of specific services.

2.88   Dutt and Ahmad further note the requirements in the Griffiths report (Griffiths, 1988) for consultation and information in the context of responding to the multi-racial nature of British society. But they comment that Black people have been largely overlooked by pre-existing consultative processes. "Carers, 'consumers', and providers should be linked into the planning and monitoring outcome processes . . . It is time that it was recognised that Black communities have developed strategies for maintaining care supports due to the failures and discrimination of service providers" (p.42).

2.89   Also, they stress the importance of knowledge and information in relation to empowerment. Language can be used as a barrier to exclude people. For example, a mother offered respite care for her child may understand "care" as meaning removal of the child for good. People need to be addressed in their own language, simple and jargon-free and the low level of public service knowledge must be remedied (Dutt and Ahmad, 1991).

2.90   Elsewhere, Arshi Ahmad has argued for use of outreach work in the places freqented by Black people (religious institutions, community centres, street markets) as a means of informing people about services (Ahmad, A, 1990). Another approach was adopted by the Black Communities Care Project at NISW which commissioned a play, *Bloodlines*, about the implications of the new legislation for individuals, to be shown to community groups (Jones, 1991). Information for consumers was also distributed by means of a booklet (Manuel, 1991).

2.91   Jones points out that consultation has become "a very tainted word" in the experience of Black people, being too often used by social services departments to confirm decisions already made, to give an appearance of change or even as a means of creating division among community groups. She quotes Arshi Ahmad on the purposes of consultation, which are:

●   to ensure that services are both accessible and appropriate;

●   to obtain expertise and knowledge the organisation lacks in order to plan and deliver services;

●   it is a crucial part of the process of accountability;

●   it is a means of recognising that services are not equitable and finding the will to address this;

●   it is a central part of policy and practice and influences both planning and complaints (Jones, 1991).

2.92   Similar issues of research and gaps in basic knowledge in relation to ethnic minorities are evident in child care. For example, in *Patterns and Outcomes* (DoH, 1990b) it is concluded that:

"The new Children Act requires consideration of a child's racial origin and culture. However, recent research reports do not provide many suggestions about how this is to be put into effect. Indeed, in many of them ethnic issues are not addressed." (p.14)

2.93   The importance of the absence of such basic information is revealed by the example of one of the studies cited (Bebbington and Miles, 1989) which identified that children with mixed racial parentage were "two and a half times as likely to enter care as white children, all other things being equal". Such findings may challenge important preconceptions, and thus highlight the need for full information.

Positive approaches to ethnic minority communities

2.94 Bandana Ahmad (1990) has used case histories to illuminate her arguments for a social work that takes full account of the strengths of Black families and communities. A "pathological framework" which relies on preconceptions of Black people as being different and presenting problems may result in inappropriate assessments and hence the failure of proferred services to resolve difficulties. Appropriate assessments imply not only an understanding of culture and language, but also the acknowledgment of the context of the family, community and society. She writes:

> "Joint ownership means joint action that is more likely to alleviate self-helplessness of the isolated individual. More importantly, joint ownership and joint action, more often than not, lead to realistic understanding of those problems which cannot be resolved completely, as neither the individual nor his or her family community have controls over the root causes of the problems". (p.14)

2.95 Arshi Ahmad makes a similar point about recognising the positive:

> "Failure to take account of the strength of Black families is equivalent to, on the one hand, operating within a framework of cultural deficit which rules out the possibility of empowerment, self help, self control and self determination of the Black client; while, on the other, it means an inability to recognise the valuable resources of potential service providers and support from the Black communities". (Ahmad, A, 1990 p.27)

2.96 Emphasising the importance of taking into account such elements of culture as religious beliefs and daily living habits, she warns against simplification and racist interpretations. Workers tend to bring their own agendas to their work, and applying their own preceptions of "cultural issues" as the all-pervasive factor affecting Black clients can result in de-skilling and faulty judgements. Examples are considering sexual abuse by a father to be "normal behaviour" in the context of a family's culture, and the needs of South Asian or Chinese girls who are in conflict with their parents (Ahmad, A, 1990).

2.97　Black social workers, suggests Bandana Ahmad (1990), have little difficulty in adopting community social work models avoiding "clientisation" of individuals, though the Black perspective of community social work has not been properly acknowledged.

2.98　The community based schemes examined by Crosbie and Vickery included two centres for ethnic minorities run predominantly by social services workers and two ethnic minority projects which had obtained funding to employ special co-ordinators, and which were therefore virtually independent. These examples indicate that automony has gains and losses. The relatively independent schemes were able to develop in their own way and expand when they found extra resources free from constraints imposed by the local authority. But they also found it more difficult than the social work run iniatives to access the departmental resources such as specialised equipment, accommodation and transport facilities.

Planning as a product of negotiation between providers, users and carers

2.99　The spirit and the letter of the community care reforms strongly support the view that planning, at whatever level, should be conducted through a process of negotiated collaboration between all the relevant "stakeholders". This is evident in the need to ascertain users' views of desirable outcomes, injunctions about enabling the independence and choice of users, and the general need to develop "needs-led" services.

2.100　The Children Act also implies that the very processes of planning and assessment must be a negotiated collaboration. A particularly strong emphasis is placed on the "empowerment" of different "users", the child, parents and members of the wider family network. Planning and assessment will, of necessity, have to be negotiated between these different "users" of the legislation.

2.101　These ideas will take time to implement as they involve attitudinal changes at all levels of service. The fear must be that, if change is too quickly urged and expected (DoH, 1985), it will lead to loss of morale and commitment. The extent of current demoralisation needs to be recognised.

2.102 The work of family centres in establishing community-based practice is described in several contexts (Smale and Bennett, 1989; Darvill and Smale, 1990; Gibbons, 1990, referred to in more detail below). Particular stress was placed in these projects on preventative work with families and development work in neighbourhood-based social networks. Management issues which need to be confronted are:

- the relationship between local management committees of family centres and other schemes and local authority hierarchies;

- the need for local management to have a high degree of autonomy or delegated responsibility if the public are to be given genuine choice in planning services and working in partnership.

2.103 The extent of the difficulties in implementing the general principle of partnership is amply illustrated in child care research. A conclusion of the research into child placements is that:

"If a partnership is to be established on a secure basis, there needs to be shared perceptions and agreement on what has gone wrong and on the more difficult area of what has to be done to improve matters. The researchers show how easy it is to be unaware of serious differences in perspective and to misinterpret actions and responses. During a recent study of child care and decision making in Northern Ireland, Kelly (HMSO, 1990) found that 'it was very difficult to find examples of social workers and parents . . . agreeing on the difficulties and working together to try and resolve them'". (DoH 1990b, G. Kelly quoted p.40)

2.104 The dominance of crisis work, associated with conflicting pressures from other services and from clients, prevents carefully negotiated planning and the effective management of workers' time (DoH, 1985 pp.6,7, 14). As a result, the differing perspectives of clients and social workers are often not recognised (p. 8); this is particularly apparent in respect of shared and differing values and attitudes (pp.12, 17), and in the devaluing of clients' potential contribution and their feelings (pp.19, 21). Even when plans are negotiated at the start of a case, planning frequently dissipates after the making of the first decision: for example, children experience unrehearsed changes of placement and worker, their discharge from care is unplanned, parents feel increasingly ignored (DoH, 1985 pp.9, 11, 13) and receive little support (p.20). Professional intervention can be disabling (Hadley et al, 1987 p.11).

2.105   Managerial and professional attention must be given to the management of time and to the enabling and empowering of users and carers (Hadley et al, 1987 p.11). The risks are that negotiation, client participation and partnership may lead to a sort of democratic laissez-faire, in which professional responsibility is abnegated, or to the endless (and frequently fruitless) search for consensus (Hadley et al, 1987 p.198). Partnership:

- requires the recognition that clients are, in certain senses, experts (Darvill and Smale, 1990 p.77; Crosbie et al, 1989 p.97);

- involves continuing two-way learning (Crosbie et al, 1989 p.103);

- is fostered by proactive activity—rather than reaction—by social workers (Crosbie et al, 1989 p.94);

- needs to be challenging and honest if it is not to lead **either** to worker's inactivity **or** to the generation of future conflicts, particularly about accountability and definitions of need and outcome (Crosbie et al, 1989 pp.156, 176–7).

Carers

2.106   Barclay, Griffiths, *Caring for People* and the guides to the Children Act all emphasise the need to support carers and recognise them as the mainstay of care in the community for all those dependent upon others, be they adults or children. *Caring for People* also stressed the need to target resources on the most needy **and** to intervene as little as possible to maintain independence (House of Commons, 1989). These three issues taken together could lead to dilemmas over the allocation of resources. (See Chapter Three). Here we need to draw attention to the relevant research findings. In their conclusions on services to elderly people Sinclair and his colleagues (1990) suggest that the success of the community care reforms may rest largely on the ability of the system to give relatively small amounts of support to maintain large numbers of people currently looked after by relatives or neighbours in the community. The research evidence on the needs of carers clearly indicates that there is a need to target resources, often in small amounts, on the support of carers of those who may not be seen by social services as "the most needy".

2.107 Levin and her colleagues carried out a detailed study of family carers of elderly people with dementia (Levin et al, 1989). They identified the enormous scale on which care is provided by sources other than statutory services. Over 80% of elderly people with dementia are cared for by family members in the old person's own home or the home of a family member. Those at home in whom the degree of dementia is severe are as seriously ill as those in institutions, and also likely to be afflicted with other mental and physical illnesses.

2.108 Big differences were identified between areas in the availability of statutory services and in take-up of benefits. Take-up of service depended heavily on whether carers referred themselves for help, and subsequently re-referred themselves. The need for action **before** the carer becomes exhausted was emphasised. There should be:

- early identification of need;

- comprehensive medical and social assessments;

- continuing back-up and reviews.

The existence of family carers was found to be a crucial factor in decisions as to whether or not elderly people with dementia require residential care. Attributes of carers (condition, level of strain, attitudes) had a major influence on whether dependents went into residential care or stayed at home.

2.109 Factors leading to strain and eventual breakdown of home care included incontinence and social restrictions for carers, but the major factors were problems of relations within the family, especially deviant behaviour of the elderly person. (See also Challis et al, 1990.) Often one carer provided most of the care, operating inside a "latent" network of the family members, neighbours, volunteers and fellow carers and the rest of the network often needed support from outside before they could integrate their contributions, and also before they could accept statutory care. The carers interviewed expressed appreciation towards those professionals who gave them recognition and the opportunity to express their feelings, and helped them to come to terms with changes (Levin et al, 1989).

Self-help groups: support workers and professionals

2.110　Sommerlad and Webb, as part of the evaluation of the Self-Help Alliance, showed how staff employed full time in CVS, SSD etc. to specialise in giving support and assistance to self-help groups (whether in voluntary or statutory agencies) provide a unique bridge encouraging two-way traffic between mainstream professionals and individuals in need. They encourage professionals in health and social services to join informal networks of self-help, and facilitate them to do this, particularly to gain access to ethnic minority communities. They also encourage user demand for statutory services (Sommerlad and Webb, 1988). Hatch and Hinton's study of Contact a Family also showed how involvement in a self-help group might not necessarily lead to a reduction in personal stress, but did lead to greater use of statutory services (Hatch and Hinton, 1986).

2.111　Sommerlad and Webb also noted how involvement of professionals in self-help networks contributed to the re-education of those professionals about their statutory services, leading in some cases to new joint services or alternative services.

2.112　Grass roots organisations with community orientated values are already welcoming the enhanced opportunities under the Community Care Act to run their own services according to their own value systems. This includes defining for themselves precisely who has what needs—people in the network as well as identified "dependent" individuals—and deciding the details of what services are offered to which people and their networks in order to empower them.

2.113　One lesson which has to be learnt is the need for professionals to avoid overloading groups with inappropriate referrals. In particular, groups find it difficult to cope with people in crisis, especially if those individuals are new to the group (Sommerlad and Webb, 1988).

Family centres

2.114　Gibbons carried out and reported on a major study of the relation-ship between statutory social services and local community activity. These important data describe the relationship between a social services department office covering an urban population of 151,000 and a network of family centres and their satellite community groups.

2.115   The study highlighted:

- how central social services workers, especially social
  workers, are less successful than local community oriented
  services in identifying need, and clearly fail to involve
  people from local networks and groups in assessment or care
  management;

- how informal networks and community groups can meet
  certain needs, and can meet some more effectively than
  centralised social services. (Details follow below). (Gibbons,
  1990)

Identifying need, and referral practice

2.116   The family projects described by Gibbons attracted significantly
more of those people in the greatest need than other people with
less need. They were involved with a quarter of the poorest
families, especially lone parents, which was equal numerically
to the SSD contact in those localities with these kinds of people,
although the scale of SSD operations was much greater.

2.117   However there was still a large shortfall since over three
quarters of high need lone parents did not use family centres: in
spite of the success of the centres in meeting certain kinds of
needs, social workers were not active in referring families to
these centres. In fact, the amount of contact between families and
family centres actually decreased during a four month period
after families came into contact with social services.

2.118   There were some resources whose take-up by families in contact
with the SSD did seem to increase. These included short-term
fostering, special childminding and marriage guidance: the
centralised and in most cases departmentally controlled resources.

2.119   The social workers studied by Gibbon did not use the centres as a
stimulus for wider involvement with community organisations
either. They were no more likely to work with volunteers or self-
help groups than staff in a control area which had a much less
extensive network of community-based organisations. However,
the work described by Macfarlane, Henderson and Higginson does
include the work of practitioners who used family centres as a
base for "outreach" work in the community (Smale and Bennett,
1989; Darvill and Smale, 1990).

2.120   Family centres may be seen as particularly appropriate vehicles
for enhancing the quality of collaboration between professional

staff and others in the community. However, the finding by Vallender (1990) that out of a sample of 352 family centres only one quarter had any parents on their management committees, gives some indication of how far there is to go in developing such collaboration and partnership.

Support from networks, and services

2.121   In the families studied by Gibbon, the core of the parents' social networks consisted of their own parents and own nuclear family (35%), followed by friends (25%). Neighbours constituted only around 3% or 4% of the networks of these families, whether they were people referred to the SSD (the referred sample) or were part of a general community sample.

2.122   The referred sample to a much greater extent than the general sample identified close family members as a major source of conflict. Neighbours provide over a quarter of the conflict relationships in both samples. When the referred sample of families were under stress, they valued emotional and social support, but especially instrumental help (child care, domestic help, money).

2.123   Where did this help come from? For families experiencing "malaise", broadly emotional distress, support received from informal sources such as family, friends and neighbours appeared the most important element in explaining improvement, rather than either formal statutory help or contact with community groups. In particular families responded to help received from friends rather than from other family members, especially their instrumental help. In this respect the emphasis may differ from elderly people, who in the Networks study wanted personal practical help from relatives or professionals, and other tasks to be done by neighbours or friends (Sinclair et al, 1988).

2.124   In fact parents receiving a statutory service, especially those in the high need group, were less likely to show improvement than those in similar need who had not been referred.

2.125   For families experiencing wider parenting problems (i.e. wider than malaise), improvement was equally likely whether they were referred for statutory help or not. There was a significant association between improvement and the number of reported contacts between families and voluntary agencies or community groups (especially playgroups, mother and toddler groups, nurseries and local child minders).

2.126 Gibbons concluded that "support of family, friends, neighbours and the use of day care, are as or more important than help received from social services or organised community groups".

2.127 The study also identified the superior role of family centres, in comparison to social services, in stimulation and support of informal networks and day care activity.

Direct and indirect care

2.128 A distinction is frequently drawn between direct and indirect social work. Direct work has been defined as work with individuals and their immediate families and networks to tackle problems which directly affect them; while indirect work is work with wider community groups and other agencies to tackle problems which affect a range of people (including the individuals involved in direct work) (Smale et al, 1988 pp.113–4). Indirect social work proved difficult for the teams studied by Sinclair et al in the face of other priorities. Obstacles included dilemmas of choice (service development versus community development); structural obstacles to decision-making within the area teams; lack of resources; and organisational difficulties caused by different boundaries of geographical areas. Positive factors were the support of senior social workers; the case review system; selection of a manageable focus; allocation of workers' time; allocation of responsibility to small groups of workers; staff skills in working with the hierarchy and other professions; and availability of volunteers (Sinclair et al, 1988).

The idea of neighbourhood care

2.129 Abrams considered neighbourhood care:

> "The idea of neighbourhood care accredits a fusion of the formal and informal, of egoism and altruism, of reciprocity and patronage, of autonomy and social control, of tradition and innovation, of self help and dependency. Such a package of antitheses is bound to be riddled with moral ambiguity and a rich mine of evaluative conflict . . . Those of us who believe in neighbourhood care are stuck with the task of defending an enterprise which devotees of simple moralities will assail from all sides. We can do so in my view only by asserting strenuously the pragmatic desirability of contradiction . . ." (Bulmer, 1986 pp.223 and 225)

2.130 Abrams' astute eye for contradiction, ambiguity and paradox is evident in his discussion of the nature of "care". It is not possible to extract a simple, generic definition from his work. A dimension of this is the subjectivity of "care".

2.131 Understanding care "involves understanding the very different meanings that care can have for different people in different social situations and different caring projects" (p.202). This is clearly a major issue when working with Black and ethnic minority groups (Ahmad, A, 1990).

2.132 Of care by neighbours he concluded:

> ". . . the long-term, arduous, time-consuming work of continuous care of an elderly or disabled person would be most unlikely to be undertaken by a neighbour unless there was added to neighbourliness some additional element such as friendship. These issues are of considerable relevance to policies to promote community care through neighbourliness". (Bulmer, 1986 p.171)

Social control and bad neighbouring

2.133 Most research on "neighbouring" has focused on positive, helping dimensions. However, Abrams recognized the "razor's edge" that divides good from bad neighbouring and the need to research this area, not least because what research there is implies "that bad neighbouring involves only a slight tipping of the relational balance that sustains good neighbouring" (Bulmer, 1986 p.32). Further study of the relationship between good and bad neighbouring would, in a sense, be a study of social control:

> "Social control can . . . be enforced through myriad forms of neighbouring such as gossip, casual conversation and informal surveillance—all of which subject individuals to purportedly collective sets of norms and expectations". (Bulmer, 1986 p.32)

2.134 Social welfare agencies are often drawn into situations in which informal social control is ineffective, and in which "bad neighbouring" is taking place. This may be the problem that has to be tackled to effect a string of "individual" referrals (Smale et al, 1988).

2.135 Development work carried out through the Community Social Work Exchange at the National Institute for Social Work revealed the degree to which many social workers had continually to wrestle with issues of social control, in contrast to many reports (e.g. Barclay, 1982 and Griffiths, 1988) which are chiefly concerned with service delivery. The authors and practitioners who contributed to the Community Social Work Exchange agreed that most, if not all, social work and social services intervention involves social control in one form or another. By this it is meant that help is being requested within a social situation in which somebody's behaviour is being defined as deviant, difficult or otherwise having unfortunate consequences on other people's well-being. Situations where, for example, elderly people are left socially isolated and at risk are by this definition as much issues of "deviance" as more obvious cases of child abuse or juvenile delinquency. The major thrust of this discussion is the necessity for those who deliver social work and social services to recognise that much of their work inevitably involves social control and intervention designed to change the way that people relate to each other. Service delivery may well be part of this intervention but often action needs to go well beyond this. Inevitably moral and political issues are raised by this awareness and the authors argue that this strengthens the need for partnership with all people in the community to define what methods and priorities social services and social work departments should adopt (Smale et al, 1988).

Change

2.136   Abrams' later work implies more than it explicitly asserts about the strategies and tactics for changing patterns of relationships which are the source of social problems. Our understanding of such patterns is improved, but there is less emphasis on what actually to do in order to change problematic situations. Take, for example, these quotations from Abrams' work, edited by Bulmer:

> "... reciprocity was in some important respects a matter of possibilities within the caring relationship which some perceived and many did not. If that conclusion was justified, it would follow that a great deal more informal care could in principle be unleashed by appropriate social policies". (Bulmer, 1986 p.10)

This "unleashing" would consist of changing people's perceptions so that they perceive the possibilities of reciprocal responses to their "giving" when at present they do not. What such change consists of, and how it is to be achieved, is by no means fully mapped out:

> "The principal obstacles to personal involvement in neighbourhood care appear to be lack of time, lack of skills,

and lack of confidence. These obstacles can quite easily be overcome by suitably modest processes of induction". (Bulmer, 1986 p.128)

"Many of the people who initially joined Good Neighbour schemes and then dropped out appeared to withdraw precisely because they did not know how to be useful." (Bulmer, 1986)

2.137   These are both examples of an implied focus of change, where helpers need assistance in matching their abilities to tasks, and help in developing the competencies needed. Many people described as "carers" do not see themselves in this way. They did not decide to take on the responsibility nor do they recognise the skills and resources they bring to bear; they "just got on with the job" when the need arose and they found themselves having to do it all. There are many similar implications for change, although they are not systematized and the processes needed to make such changes are not themselves at the foreground in Abrams' work. The need for change in social networks is also discussed by Smale et al (1988); examples of work undertaken by social workers to achieve such change are discussed by Cooper and others in Darvill and Smale (1990).

Loneliness

2.138   Abrams identifies and analyses the complex problem of loneliness. For example:

"Childlessness, whether actual or in effect, was in itself a crucial source of isolation and of the resulting need for neighbourhood care. The world of the clients of neighbourhood care was not at all a world of densely woven informal relationships with neighbourhood care. Helpers simply added on to social contact with family, friends and neighbours. Though the most significant contacts were with other members of the family, it was distinctively a world of significant isolation from informal care." (Bulmer, 1986 p.167)

2.139   The nature of loneliness, isolation and the differing kinds of dependency needs which are thus unmet, require detailed and specific understanding. If a person is lonely because they do not see their children as regularly as they would like, there is no guarantee that that particular quality of loneliness will be much affected by other forms of social contact. Nor will it necessarily be affected by the provision of services.

2.140 Isolation, in the sense of individuals not having the kinds of social relationships they need, is the central social problem revealed by the PSSRU work. However, this is not always obvious. For example, "immobility" is framed as a problem, but not necessarily seen as requiring the involvement of social work agencies. Such agencies get involved when a person's mobility is impaired and they lack the necessary relationships to help them with this.

2.141 The most physically dependent people on the Neighbourhood Care Scheme were "bedfast". Frequently, unless such people have a great deal of family support, they are unable to remain at home (Bulmer, 1986 p.41). Being "bedfast" may be experienced as a personal problem, but it becomes a social problem because of "isolation" or the absence of the necessary personal relationships. This is true for all the problems addressed by the case management schemes.

2.142 Isolation and loneliness are seen as major contributory factors in behaviour which is problematic for that person's network. For example:

> "... one important element which was evident early on was the extent to which isolation, understimulation or sensory deprivation could magnify the impact of the dementing condition." (Bulmer, 1986 p.44)

Local planning of schemes

2.143 Crosbie and Vickery (1989) found that most schemes came about as a result of staff's experience with individual clients and their local knowledge of resources, rather than a systematic assessment of need. Information was lacking about the needs of those who had not been referred to social services. Thus it could be guessed that a small town would contain more than enough potential users to justify a day club, but research (Sokolovsky, 1989) supports the desirability of proper assessments of the needs of ethnic minority groups, due to the variability of the type of provision acceptable to different populations (Crosbie and Vickery, 1989 p.82). Those area offices most committed to the development of community resources were most likely to create means of assessing needs and resources, including obtaining assistance from external researchers (Crosbie and Vickery, 1989 p.140). Community workers were much more aware than social workers of needs that had not impinged on the area office.

2.144   The availability of resources varied greatly between areas. In
        some there was a good fund of groups and voluntary organisations
        willing to contemplate new work and good liaison arrangements
        to discuss need in general; yet some possible sources of energy
        might be overlooked. This was also true of poor neighbourhoods,
        lacking basic amenities and social cohesion and characterised by
        social isolation, crime and fewer formal voluntary organisations.
        In such localities those area offices with explicit policies on
        working with local communities were involved with a wider
        range of informal groups, including church groups and minority
        ethnic groups, and therefore understood more accurately what
        resources were available. Workers in the Dinnington project
        increased significantly the contacts they made in the community
        (Bayley et al, 1989 pp.112 on). The researchers suggest that,
        apart from special enquiries, observing and recording unmet needs
        is a responsibility of area staff, and they have an obligation to
        enquire into clients' social networks and to broaden their
        knowledge of local resources (Crosbie and Vickery, 1989 pp.85–6).

Assessment and care management

2.145   The community care reforms seek to ensure that the processes of
        assessment and care management include:

        ● full assessment of the user's circumstances in the round;

        ● the design of packages of care in agreement with users, carers
          and relevant agencies, and feedback into the wider planning
          process of any identified shortfalls in provision;

        ● implementation, monitoring and revision of the agreed
          package of care.

2.146   Within this broad framework, particular emphasis has been
        given to the separation of assessment from service provision, and
        the purchase of services from the provision of services. Care
        management, as such, is not defined within the framework of the
        Children Act reforms, but the processes of assessment and service
        provision are based on the same basic principles of assessment in
        the round, user and carer involvement, and explicit ongoing
        monitoring and revision of plans and agreements.

Assessment and care management for elderly people

2.147   Professionals typically have a controlling role in the allocation
        of services, despite the opportunity of old people and their carers

to refer themselves initially. Social services departments might be seen as a means of meeting the needs of professionals who do not wish to deal themselves with certain problems, such as the emotional or boring problems of doctors' patients. They can appear to be more effective in "managing" these problems, and people's concern over particular people, than they are of meeting the needs of their identified "clients". In practice the identity of the customer is often debatable, even if "the client" is all too easily assumed to be a single individual (Smale et al, 1991). Most referrals originate with other professionals and therefore they control definitions of need. This may be one reason, Sinclair et al (1990) suggest, for the alleged fragmentation of services and their lack of responsiveness to their consumers. The key advocates of and referrers for standard social services are general practitioners, social workers, hospital staff and health visitors, all of whom have to provide a mixture of services and respond to an assortment of demands. These professionals also have to defend "their" services and in turn encounter defensive attitudes from other professionals and hence may be uncertain about the quality of other services (Sinclair et al, 1990 pp.157–8). One interesting feature of the Dinnington project with its emphasis on easy open access was a dramatic increase in self-referrals by elderly people. Over a two-year period the referrals went up nearly seven times, so that over four in ten of the elderly population on average had contact with the local office in the course of a year (Bayley et al, 1989 pp.108–110).

2.148 Among the research results cited are:

- principal problems dealt with at referral arise from the **personal and social consequences** of ill health and disability, but the main focus of what social workers do is upon investigation and assessment of an individual, and thereafter upon the mobilisation of resources;

- long-term social work is more likely than short-term social work to be concerned with sustaining clients and solving problems, and involves contact with other professionals, relatives, neighbours and friends;

- in seven out of ten long-term cases involving an elderly person someone expected the social worker to move the client to a safer setting, and there was quite often a disagreement between the "client" and others about the need for such a move.

2.149   From the above it is reasoned that long-term social work with elderly people is predominantly concerned with situations where a routine response is difficult, and is characterised by the seriousness of the decisions to be made, the types of clients (frail or "difficult to help") the range of services contacted and interests considered, and the likelihood of conflict over decisions (Sinclair et al, 1990 p.147).

2.150   Discharge from hospital is one route to the assistance of social services. The term "blocked beds" describes situations in which people are medically fit to go home, but remain in hospital because appropriate accommodation and support are not available elsewhere. One study showed the effects of an increasing emphasis on rapid discharge from acute beds and reductions in long-stay hospital beds for elderly people. This brought about increasing use of the private residential sector, including private nursing homes, and in a few places residential assessment centres and "home from hospital" schemes. Since hospital discharge was a key point in the allocation of services to elderly people, and not a point at which the social needs of elderly patients were given high priority, improvements in the process of discharge were urgently needed (Sinclair et al, 1990 p.155).

2.151   Systems of assessment and referral are disjointed. Professionals may experience conflict between their wish to act as advocate for clients and the need to conserve scarce resources and they may not control or even be seen as entitled to recommend the service they believe is required. GPs often know little of patients' social problems, while on the other hand home-helps and district nurses know individuals better but do not take key roles in referral. Social workers often do not consider medical problems and multi-disciplinary assessment is rare (Sinclair et al, 1990 p.220).

Assessing individuals' networks

2.152   The study by Sinclair et al of elderly people living alone suggested that assessment should take account of the clients as individuals, the client's network and the subjective environment, i.e. the views and feelings of the clients, carers, agency resource-holders and other professionals about the current situation and what should be done about it.

2.153   The development workers found that social workers were predominantly concerned with the degree to which clients were "at risk". So in order to assist decisions about staying at home or moving to residential care workers examined depression, mental confusion, the client's failure to behave prudently, the effects of living alone while being physically ill or disabled, and environmental factors such as trip hazards or poor heating.

2.154 In assessing clients' networks workers had to consider whether adequate physical care was offered; whether there was sufficiently frequent contact with the client to ensure safety; and whether to give the client a sense of social and emotional well-being. Also to be taken into account were the degree and nature of the carers' physical and emotional stress, the degree to which carers were supporting or sabotaging the client's aims and the likely durability of the client's networks (Sinclair et al, 1988).

2.155 Often there were just too few people in the network to cover all that was needed. The client's safety was clearly more easily ensured when the level of physical care was high and was being given by a group of carers who, between them, might see the client three to four times a day. It was badly met for those who, under the prevailing policy, did not warrant (or could not be allocated) more than two hours of home help twice a week, did not have a daily district nurse and did not have a neighbour popping in or a relative visiting more than weekly. These networks were particularly deficient as far as surveillance was concerned, but were also likely to be deficient in providing companionship and emotional support (Sinclair et al, 1988 p.151).

2.156 The importance of assessing individuals' networks is also underlined by much child care research, along with evidence that such network dimensions are often not fully addressed in assessment and practice generally (Department of Health, 1990b):

> "Family links are seldom given much consideration. As a result, circumstantial barriers to access may go unrecognised and little practical help is offered to encourage parents' visits. When links wither, chances of the child's return home are diminished." (p.10, para 4)

2.157 Similarly Packman et al (1986) are quoted as saying:

> "Assessments accurately reflected the facts of each family situation and also shared some parental perceptions of what the problems were. Where they were sometimes weak was in their exploration of kin and neighbourhood networks as potential sources of help . . .". (DoH, 1985 p.13)

2.158   This perspective is maintained in the more recent research. For example, a study by Bebbington and Miles (reported in Department of Health, 1990b p.6) of 2,500 children admitted to care concluded that:

> ". . . it is probably not only the poverty of single parents but also their lack of available social supports which makes their children more liable to need looking after away from home."

2.159   Studies of young people leaving care also highlight the importance of such network links, and the need to identify and remedy deficits in such links. (For example, Stein and Carey, 1986; Wedge, unpublished.) A conclusion drawn from some of these studies is that:

> "The well-being of young care leavers depends not just on practical matters such as housing and employment, vital though they are . . . It is a useful, if salutary, exercise to consider what relationships and resources are available to each young person moving into independent living arrangements. What links do they have with parents, siblings, other relatives? With past carers and social workers? With peers? With people in the community? To whom can they turn for emotional support, for advice or companionship?" (Department of Health, 1990b p.12)

Assessment and the social worker's role

2.160   The development workers who collaborated with Sinclair et al concluded that there was little scope for any great reduction in workers' caseloads and that assessments in particular could profitably be awarded more time. Workers were criticised for seeking limited information on the need for services and the client's willingness to accept them, rather than explaining how clients were experiencing their predicament. On the whole clients were not perceived as potential resources and their capacity to resume a role or find a new one was not assessed. In several cases workers were considered not to have explored networks thoroughly. Most workers were too remote from key carers, including home helps, either to use them as assessors or to understand sufficiently their need for support. There was also insufficient contact with other professionals for adequate joint assessments of some of the clients with complex medical problems. Even when there was obvious conflict between clients and carers or between clients/carers and the agency, workers tended to avoid or ignore it. Resource gaps were not always recorded in order to develop broader perspectives.

2.161　So lack of time reinforced a crisis/service oriented approach that turned the social worker mainly into a mobilizer of scarce resources. The ability to define problems in as many ways as possible and to discover alternative resources was exercised by only a few workers—in general time needed to discover new resources for individual cases was simply not available.

2.162　Two models of practice were described, the "social worker as discoverer/creator of resources" and the "social worker as mobiliser of scarce resources". Teams agreed that they needed to move towards the former role. The several resource gaps then identified included home nursing and night-sitters, transport, befrienders and means of linking housebound people with each other (Sinclair et al, 1988 p.160).

Care management and the guidelines

2.163　The separation proposed between assessors of need and providers of services will need to take account of the traditional integration of the roles in professional education and practice, and the likely reluctance of professional workers to be forced into one or other of these roles. The risks involved in this enforced separation are:

- that assessment will be removed from the reality of what services can actually be provided within the resources available;

- that assessment may become insensitive and managerial;

- that social workers will feel they are being further deprofessionalised;

- that provisions will be based exclusively and unimaginatively on the ideology and vision (however limited) of one assessor.

2.164　On the other hand, the emphasis in legislation on a bottom-up contribution to assessment could be a safeguard against these dangers, provided users and carers are defined as joint care-managers or some other way is found of incorporating input from carers. (See Smale et al, 1993 for further discussion of these issues).

2.165   Care managers will need to be constantly aware of the volatility
         of informal care, the vulnerability of informal networks, and the
         limitations of consistency among informal carers (Bayley et al,
         1989 pp.49, 180).

2.166   Effective care management will therefore require skills in the
         following areas of practice:

         •   planning strategies of intervention **with** service-users, based
             on specific information about the availability, nature and
             reliability of informal networks of resources;

         •   defining the specific tasks to be undertaken;

         •   identifying who can undertake particular tasks, negotiating
             their agreement to do so, and informing each of the
             complementary activities of others;

         •   ensuring the means whereby all the efforts will be co-
             ordinated and monitored (Hadley et al, 1987 p.146).

2.167   The Children Act clarifies and underlines the range of ways in
         which local authorities are responsible for ensuring that other
         people and organisations appropriately discharge their
         responsibilities for care of children. This responsibility on local
         authorities will be carried out by those engaged in the four broad
         activities outlined above. For example, the Act asserts that:

         "Care and supervision orders place such important
         responsibilities on local authorities that it is left to them to
         decide, taking into account the circumstances identified in their
         investigation, whether or not to apply for an order. Moreover,
         it will be for them to decide what other sources may be
         provided to the family which might preclude any order being
         made."

         This clearly puts the local authority staff into the position of
         planning and managing a "package of care" for children in need.

2.168   Smale et al (1988) have suggested certain processes essential to
         effective teamwork and to the effectiveness of departmental
         organisation. Though not directly concerned with "care
         management" as defined in the guidelines to the legislation,
         their suggestions could well be used as a definition of the
         responsibilities of the care manager additional to the
         diagnosis/assessment of the individual case.

2.169   We have identified the following issues based on the basic
        assumptions and values held by those involved:

        ● patterns of existing relationships and activities;

        ● criteria of a good outcome;

        ● procedures for future monitoring/evaluation;

        ● implications for organisational development and relevant
          social/community changes.

What is care?

2.170   The research definition of "care" used by Challis et al is
        contained within discussion of direct and indirect care, but a
        difficulty is that some of the central activities engaged in by care
        managers in the schemes are not usefully described as "care" at
        all. It may be unhelpful to describe this often complex process of
        change in an interpersonal network as "care". For example:

        > "Sometimes in working with carers a great deal of effort had
        > to be put into undoing the original support network and
        > encouraging friends and relatives to withdraw". (Challis et al,
        > 1990 p.47)

2.171   Analysis of the nature of this change and control task, and of the
        knowledge and skills required to carry it out effectively, is
        hindered by the implicit assumption that it must be either direct
        or indirect "care".

2.172   A dimension of "indirect care", the creation of "new" resources by
        changing existing provision in some way is clearly important, but
        the process involved is under-described. For example, a social
        activity group around meal times was set up in a sheltered
        housing unit to provide stimulation, companionship and activity,
        but the process of creating this innovation was not described or
        analysed. The negotiations necessary within the institution, the
        changing of staff roles, and the monitoring of its impact on other
        residents are all dimensions of a change process which will be
        important factors in the success or otherwise of the innovation:
        that is, the creation of new resources by changing existing
        practices, but more analysis of this would be useful.

Process of intervention

2.173   The Gateshead scheme emphasises the importance of an
        integrated process of care management and service delivery. How

the workers relate to those they are working with is seen as crucial. For example:

> "Although very often the tasks required of helpers would be essentially practical in nature, it was the way in which the approach was made to the elderly person that proved important". (Challis et al, 1990 p.39)

> "The way in which help was offered in the approach of both the case manager and the helpers appeared to be crucial to effective outcomes. Often a pattern of one-to-one communication had to be resurrected as elderly people had often been talked over on the assumption that they were unable to understand". (Challis et al, 1990 p.45)

2.174   Process in the sense of the creating of a synthesis or integration of different responses is shown to be crucial. In comparing the responses of the scheme and the standard provision, the main flaw of the latter is seen as its failure to create a process of integration within the usual responses. It is concluded that:

> "What is important is that it illustrates how the outcome of care using the conventional range of services may be unsatisfactory even when the agencies are actively and constructively involved." (Challis et al, 1990 p.51)

What is "care management"?

2.175   Challis et al make a distinction between "administrative" and "complete" case management. They write:

> "It is possible to define a rather limited form of case management—described here as "administrative" case management—where service arrrangements and coordination are seen as the central tasks. The other tasks of case management such as counselling, dealing with psychological stresses and tensions arising from caring or providing advice to families would be undertaken by persons other than the case manager ... An underlying weakness in the "administrative" model of case management is the failure to recognise the nature of the responsibilities and decisions which have to be made by the case manager." (Challis et al, 1990 p.15)

2.176   It is clear throughout the book describing the Gateshead project that "complete" case management is what the authors think case management essentially is. It is also clear that this approach differs significantly from that being promoted in the white paper, subsequent legislation and accompanying implementation papers. The argument of Challis et al is clear, and well illustrated, but it does not go far enough either in its theoretical formulation or its practice implications.

2.177   The white paper and the subsequent implementation papers argued for a separation of "assessment" and "service delivery", and for a separation of "purchasing" and "provision". The argument of Challis et al is that these separations are not feasible either theoretically or in practice. To enforce them will be to enforce an "administrative" model of case management (or care management as it is now called). Implementation of the complete model of care management cannot be achieved through these separations.

2.178   The implementation documentation clearly asserts the need for "a progressive separation of assessment from service provision . . ." and "a shift of influence from those providing to those purchasing services". However, the experience of the Gateshead project clearly questions the viability of these separations, particularly through arguing that "assessment" is a continuous process intimately interwoven with a range of direct and indirect work with the network of people involved with the "user" or "client". In the Gateshead experience assessment is not a single, or even episodic, administrative event. The authors write:

> "Neither the process of assessment nor of care packaging can be considered as a one-off activity. They are dynamic and build continuously on earlier work and require responses to changing circumstances and previously concealed problems". (Challis et al, 1990 p.35)

2.179   In addition, the work of the care manager is more diverse and complex than the "purchasing of services". It is clear that the care manager has to engage in very diverse tasks, at least some of which are the kinds of tasks traditionally viewed as aspects of "service provision". For example, Challis et al write:

> "Not uncommonly, the package of care consisted of mobilising and reorganising the input of existing services . . . This often required patient, tactful negotiations . . . Neighbours, family and friends sometimes preferred not to commit themselves to undertaking certain activities at particular times of the day . . . Fine judgements were required about when and how it was necessary to intervene in family support to improve the quality

of care without interfering unreasonably in the lives and relationships of others ..." (Challis et al, 1990 p.32)

2.180   The characteristics of what PSSRU call "complete" case management often typify work described in the Community Social Work Exchange literature. For example, the response of the Earls Court team to Ivan, a man with a history of severe mental illness, involved a complex interweaving of standard service provision: individual counselling; efforts to change relationships between Ivan, his neighbours and friends; clarification of different agency responsibilities; prior development of voluntary resources etc. (A. Cooper in Darvill and Smale, 1990). The complexity of what is actually involved in creating this "package of care" and "managing" it, reinforces and elaborates the PSSRU argument against the over-simplicity of the "administrative" model of care management. Other similar examples may be found in the CSWE literature, for example, Darvill and Smale, 1990 Chapter 6; Smale and Bennett, 1989 Chapter 4.

2.181   It is evident from the PSSRU studies, both in Gatehead and the earlier Kent material, that a central dimension of the task is to bring about changes in the way people relate to each other, and that often this means getting people to do things they might not "freely" have chosen to do. That is, social work staff are inevitably involved in aspects of "social control". It is obfuscating and perverse simply to describe such activity by the care manager as "care", or "service provision".

2.182   For example, Challis et al write:

"On some occasions it was necessary to deal with considerable conflict in an informal care network, arising from misperceptions between elderly person and carer, and attempting to resolve problems of hidden stress, guilt and difficulties in relationships. On other occasions work involved shifting the balance of demands within family groups to avoid polarisation of care on one individual ... Sometimes in working with carers a great deal of effort had to be put into undoing the original support network and encouraging friends and relatives to withdraw." (Challis et al, 1990 p.47)

Assessment

2.183   Both the PSSRU studies mentioned argue for the importance of seeing assessment as being as much a continuous process as a single event. It is argued that the assessment process has at least three elements:

"1 The eligibility screening judgement . . .

2 The initial assessment and problem specification . . .

3 Reassessment and re-evaluation of the initial formulation."

2.184   Assessment is "comprehensive". It includes:

"... the elderly person's physical and mental health, their attitude and outlook, and environmental and social circumstances, as well as their views of their most pressing problems and desired solutions ... The evaluation of risk ... The identification of retained abilities or strengths ..." (Challis et al, 1990 p.29)

Care managers

2.185   Both the Kent and Gateshead schemes were based on a single worker who undertook all the core tasks of case management. The Gateshead book contains a list of "Case Managers' activities and skills" (Challis et al, 1990 p.9). There is also an analysis of the activities engaged in by case managers in the Health and Social Care Scheme. These were broken down into the categories of direct work with clients; work with the informal network; work with scheme helpers; and work with the formal network (Challis et al, 1990 p.70). This discussion concludes:

"Once again it is clear that the case management role is far more complex than an administrative role and requires the case manager to deploy a wide range of skills". (Challis et al, 1990 p.75)

2.186   One further complexity with regard to care management is the overlap with contract management, if practice is to be flexible and effective. This overlap derives from the need to treat aspects of assessment and care management as being located at different points on a continuum. One way this continuum is already manifesting itself is in the emergence of two stages of assessment, one carried out by the SSD and the other by a providing agency, for example the residential home or Crossroads Care Attendant (CCA) scheme. The statutory care manager identifies priority clients and allocates the level of budget, but then hands over responsibility for detailed assessment and ongoing reviews and reassessments to the provider, who is contracted accordingly. A key aspect of the care manager's role thereafter is to monitor and evaluate compliance with the contract.

2.187 For example, grass roots organisations with community-oriented values are already welcoming the enhanced opportunities under the CCA to run their own services according to their own value-systems, including defining for themselves who precisely is in need—the network as well as the individual, for example—and deciding the details of what services are offered to individuals and their networks in order to empower them.

2.188 There is a further point that although specialisation is not desirable at the screeening stage, which needs to be local and accessible, nor even at the first stage of assessment, specialisation is desirable at the second stage of assessment/provision if services are to be in a position to bind together effective interorganisational networks of voluntary/community/self-help groups who identify with a particular issue or need.

2.189 This links to debates about integrating the work of different professionals. If provision is passed over to voluntary/community/independent organisations they can build their own multi-professional paid staff teams, unconstrained by traditional statutory boundaries, e.g. MIND mental health services, very local day/residential units for people with learning difficulties run by local associations employing social workers, nurses, CPNs, teachers, etc. The argument that if you specialise locally you dissipate staff into lone rangers no longer holds. People who would have been loners in their separate statutory agencies or sub-units can come together into viable specialist multi-disciplinary local teams.

2.190 There is no evidence from either scheme of inter- or intra-agency conflicts requiring management by the case manager. The multi-disciplinary team described in the Health and Social Care Scheme appears to have run very smoothly.

Combining value for money and monitoring quality of provision, having regard for users' choices

2.191 The community care reforms emphasise the need to ensure "value for money", while at the same time emphasising the importance of principles of quality assurance and respect for clients' wishes and choices. However, reconciling these sets of principles in practice may be more complicated than it might seem at first sight.

2.192   A major aspect of the "complication" alluded to above is the "social control" dimensions of "care in the community", most evident in the Children Act. What is to count as "good quality provision" may vary according to who is making the judgement. The parent whose child has been removed, the child, and other professionals involved, may all have different perceptions and criteria of "quality". Paying regard to "users' choices" means paying regard to possible conflicts of choice within a network of "users". Some safeguards against local authorities being judges of their own quality of provision have been strengthened under the Act, for example the use of powers of the guardian ad litem, and the requirement to appoint an "independent visitor" to children under certain circumstances.

2.193   These issues are particularly important in relationship to people in ethnic minorities. Definitions of adequate care will vary between ethnic groups, as is acknowledged in *Caring for People* (House of Commons, 1989). Action needs to be taken to question and resolve the problems concerning institutional racism, such as why it is that Black groups typically receive less services and yet tend to be over-represented as recipients of the social control activities of social services departments (Black Perspectives Exchange, 1990).

2.194   If monitoring and evaluating "value for money" were easy, there would have been a great deal more research in this field, both for medicine and for social work. The action-research available offers a few pointers towards unravelling the methodological complexities:

● "Value for money" policies will not be implemented unless they are related piecemeal to specific strategies and activities. This is partly due to the tension between professional workers and their bureaucracies (DoH, 1985 p.18), and partly because different strategies/activities/ client groups may require the formulation of different criteria.

● Because of ambiguous public and political attitudes concerning the right to intervene, we need to recognise that workers often adopt a "wait and see" stance (DoH, 1985 p.18), and sometimes feel helpless to intervene even when they recognise that they should (DoH, 1985 p.21).

- If we take seriously the choices and opinions of service users, we need to bear in mind the complications surrounding the use of "satisfaction" as a criterion of outcome (Bayley, 1989 p.148). Paradoxically, clients sometimes seem less appreciative of locally-based services than of traditional forms of intervention (Bayley, 1989 p.153). Similarly, workers and clients may differently evaluate the same kinds of intervention (Bayley, 1989 p.154).

- There are somewhat different views among researchers concerning the base-lines of monitoring and evaluation. Thus, Hadley advocates two contexts: by department and by local team (Hadley, 1987 pp.222–6); Bayley suggests as baselines, the workers' roles and styles of intervention (Bayley, 1989 pp.119–120). Bayley's levels of intervention are the individual, the family, the group, the network and the neighbourhood; and he identifies six roles—therapist, teacher/counsellor, broker, advocate, resource developer, consultant to networks. Any evaluations would therefore be related to thirty dimensions of practice—a realistic but somewhat more sophisticated approach than services may be willing to adopt.

- Smale and Tuson offer a more manageable matrix on the dimensions of direct-indirect work and service delivery— change agent, a matrix which additionally encompasses the extent of collaboration and the allocation of tasks (Smale and Tuson, 1988 p.16). Additionally, they list certain "core competencies" of social work practices which would, variously, be measurable (pp.25 et seq): viz the ability to negotiate partnerships and collaborative practices; resolving problem-retention mechanisms in local networks/social care planning; empathy; collating and ordering social data; inter-personal relationships; ability to be appropriately challenging and confrontational; ability to help others to define and redefine their roles and situations.

The skills of assessment and care management are discussed further in the companion report to this volume (Smale et al, 1993).

- In evaluating whether work has been both effective and efficient, Darvill and Smale (1990 p.18) suggest the following monitoring and quality-control criteria:

there should be early warning mechanisms of cases at risk;

users and carers should have ready access to provisions and adequate information about them;

plans should be jointly negotiated;

there should be appropriate local participation in the provisions recommended;

plans should be co-ordinated;

so far as is compatible with issues of equity, resources should be locally managed.

Devolved budgeting

2.195   The research reviewed supports Griffiths (1988) and *Caring for People* (House of Commons, 1989) in recommending that decisions about resource allocation should be devolved to those with most contact with, and thus knowledge of, users' circumstances.

2.196   For example, in the research on community care schemes in Kent and Gateshead the devolution of budgets to the case manager is seen as a crucial factor in fostering innovation and user-sensitive services:

> "The evidence of several case management services would indicate that control over resources has been a key factor in enabling case managers to respond more effectively to the individual needs of clients". (Challis et al, 1990 p.13)

2.197   Causal connection between devolved budgeting and better quality service is not very clearly proven by this research. There are many possible factors involved: for example, in both the Kent and Gateshead projects, the workers carry smaller caseloads than that of the "control" groups, but the influence of this factor on improved practice is not clearly distinguished from other factors, including that of devolved budgeting.

2.198   However, in *Bridging Two Worlds*, Sinclair et al (1988) found that those with most knowledge of users were divorced from resource allocation, and concluded that services could be more effective and sensitive to users' needs were this not the case.

2.199   Eight services not organised from area offices were studied by Sinclair and his colleagues (1988) in their study of social work and the elderly living at home. High levels of satisfaction were reported with GPs' community nursing services, chiropody, meals on wheels, clubs, volunteers, old people's welfare organisations and churches. Problems included a lack of resources. The district nursing, bath attendant, meals on wheels and chiropody services were criticised for spending too little time delivering the service or visiting too infrequently or unpredictably. Variability in the standards of workers was commented on, and problems of access to clubs or churches included transport difficulties and shyness. General practitioners were key referrers for elderly clients but seemed to vary considerably in their willingness to consider social needs or refer for them. Increased resources, flexibility, use of aids, improved training and supervision and increasing contacts between social services and primary health care team members would all improve efficiency in statutory services.

2.200   The study emphasised the value of the role played by the home help service. Many clients would have found it difficult, if not impossible, to exist in the community without it and it was a lifeline for many housebound clients. Benefits were both practical and social. From the point of view of the clients, home helps had four advantages in comparison with neighbours. They were more likely to go to the housebound, whereas in this sample neighbours were as likely to visit the ambulant as the housebound. Also, they could be asked to undertake practical tasks regularly without the clients necessarily feeling indebted to them. The service might be improved by improving turnover and reliability, by training or supervision procedures taking account of some of the basic techniques required, by development of a more intensive service for a small number of disabled clients, development of schemes for dealing with heavy domestic work and development of the routine surveillance role of home helps (Sinclair et al, 1988 p.96).

2.201   The development workers in the same study found four reasons why social workers were involved with elderly people:

●   to provide occasional help to a small number of clients with circumscribed problems who needed to be able to call on a social worker they knew;

●   to assess whether clients with pervasive problems could remain in the community and then either to arrange support to enable them to do so, or to apply for sheltered housing or residential care and help clients to prepare for and manage the move;

- to reassure carers of elderly clients at risk and with pervasive problems that a social worker was in touch and willing to take responsibility and, if necessary, action;

- to carry out roles that required authority and which neighbours and others were in no position to play (for example, to confront clients with the probable consequences of their behaviour or mediate in disputes over whether a client should move). These roles were typically required in cases where the clients had pervasive problems and difficult personalities.

2.202   In a small number of cases social workers were visiting simply on the grounds of the client's loneliness or because of the requirement to visit old people on the housing list for sheltered housing; neither of these were considered sufficient reasons for social work involvement (Sinclair et al, 1988 pp.145–6).

Local knowledge and payments

2.203   Abrams identified the central importance of payment for certain kinds of carers in certain kinds of social networks. He wrote:

"The Stonegate case showed how payment could harness neighbourly resources that through force of circumstances would not otherwise have been available, while also generating more informal help to the extent that it encouraged kin and neighbours to offer support to the formal help being given". (Bulmer, 1986 p.212)

2.204   He noted that in regard to payment "a distinctively working class pattern of care was in fact dependent on it and could flourish on the basis of it" (Bulmer, 1986, p.212).

2.205   Localised understanding of what kinds and degrees of payment are necessary for what kinds of care in different situations is thus essential.

Chapter Three
Implications of the Research for Management and Practice

Introduction: how people are cared for in the community

3.1   There are already something like 3.7 million "care managers" in Great Britain, none of whom are employed to care by social services departments, or anybody else. This figure does not include those who manage the care of their children.

3.2   Griffiths opened his analysis of community care with this basic statement about "The Role of the State":

> "Publicly provided services constitute only a small part of the total care provided to people in need. Families, friends, neighbours and other local people provide the majority of care in response to needs which they are uniquely well placed to identify and respond to. This will continue to be the primary means by which people are enabled to live normal lives in community settings. The proposals take as their starting point that this is as it should be, and that the first task of publicly provided services is to support and where possible strengthen these networks of carers. Public services can help by identifying such actual and potential carers, consulting them about their needs and those of the people they are caring for, and tailoring the provision of extra services (if required) accordingly.

> "The second task of the publicly provided services is to identify where these caring networks have broken down, or cannot meet the needs, and decide what public services are desirable to fill the gap." (Griffiths, 1988 p.5).

3.3   We take this definition of the role of public services as a starting point. It seems to us that it is all too easy for this perception to slip from the front of people's minds and for professional services to creep into centre stage. This happens whether services are provided by paid employees or volunteers of service organisations, whether public, voluntary sector, not-for-profit or private. A major change in our thinking is necessary to keep in mind the scale of **"normal"** care in the community and just how peripheral social services sometimes are.

3.4 Although the point is well known, it is important to restate the position within which formal care has to be located. In 1985 one adult in seven was providing care and one in five households contained a carer. In these statistics, taken from Green's (1988) analysis of *Informal Carers: General Household Survey, 1985,* unless otherwise stated, "carers" are defined as "people who were looking after, or providing some regular service for, a sick, handicapped or elderly person living in their own home or in another household; carers of children unless handicapped, are thus excluded from these figures."

3.5 There were six million carers overall in Great Britain. About 1.4 million devoted at least twenty hours per week to caring, of whom a quarter had looked after their dependent for at least ten years; 3.7 million carried the main responsibility for looking after someone: the care managers mentioned above.

3.6 Most carers looked after one person, but one fifth looked after more than one. Among carers whose dependents were outside the household, about one quarter helped two or more people. Four out of five carers were looking after someone related to them. Two in five were looking after one or both parents. Nearly one half lived within a few minutes walk of their dependent. Among carers looking after someone in the household, nearly one half devoted at least fifty hours per week to caring. The majority of carers whose dependents were outside the household spent under ten hours per week on caring activities.

3.7 Nearly one in five carers had looked after the same dependent for at least ten years. One quarter of carers currently devoting twenty hours or more per week to caring had looked after their dependent for at least ten years.

3.8 Many of the carers who were devoting long hours to caring had other responsibilities in addition to their caring role. Substantial proportions were in poor health themselves, with about one half of those aged 45 or over reporting a longstanding illness.

3.9 Women were more likely to be carers than men but the difference was not very marked: 15% of all women were carers, as compared with 12% of all men. But women were more likely than men to carry the main responsibility, either alone or with secondary support. This difference between the sexes was particularly marked among those caring for sick or handicapped children in the household, with 25% of the women coping singlehandedly compared with 8% of men. More women than men were carers of children: 95% of single parent families were headed by women (Graham, 1984).

3.10 Nearly two thirds of carers carried the main responsibility for the care of a dependent, either alone or jointly with someone else. About one quarter reported that no-one else helped. Only about one half of carers had dependents who received regular visits from health or social services or from voluntary groups. "Regular" was defined as at least once per month. Of these visitors 43% were health professionals while only 6% were social workers, 23% home-helps, 7% meals-on-wheels and 4% voluntary workers (Green, 1988).

3.11 "Something like nine-tenths of the care given to those who in various ways cannot fend for themselves in our society is given by spouses, parents, children and other kin... The ideal of domiciliary care proclaimed by the vast majority of those actually and prospectively in need of care is in effect a blunt preference for the family." (Bulmer, 1986 p.233)

3.12 Thus the heart of care in the community is care by kin. Improving care requires supporting and sustaining this commitment and building viable additions and alternatives. Improving the efficiency and effectiveness of services will largely depend upon close collaboration between all the agencies and organisations who provide services: partnerships between health, housing and social services, between public, voluntary and private sectors need to be developed at all levels of organisation. But even this will not be enough to implement the proposed reforms. Providing dependent people and their carers with more independence, autonomy and choice requires at least three parties to any of these collaborative relationships: any two or more agencies and their users.

3.13 Much of the research and development work reviewed here was carried out with practitioners and managers who shared at least some of the major assumptions that underpin the proposed reforms. Their experience is then particularly relevant. Care in the community does not have to be reinvented but much of it has to be renegotiated with the major participants: those requiring services, their users and the other people involved.

3.14   The research and development work illustrates the significance of supporting and working with carers and how the potential for others in the community to share in these tasks can be developed through the resourcing of appropriate services, as defined by users from all the different sectors of the community. Working in partnership with citizens and other agencies to develop a range of resources in the community is required to make choice a reality and will be an essential dimension of the social work task. Linking up with, and where appropriate, supporting and initiating "self-help" organisations and other community based projects are examples of the way that resources can be expanded through action with those who care in the community. These are crucial tasks for social services professionals.

3.15   Particular attention will need to be paid to address imbalances in the distribution of resources to different ethnic and minority groups. Black people can experience "triple jeopardy": they suffer the effects of racism; are disadvantaged in housing, health, employment and pensions; and services are not tailored to their general and specific needs.

The focus of professional services and intervention

The social situation as a unit of assessment

3.16   **People's social circumstances, and specifically the availability of care from their personal relationships are more significant indicators of the services they need than their individual characteristics.**

3.17   The social situation is the appropriate unit of assessment: this includes local and cultural expectations about "normal" patterns of care and support, the "clients'" and the "carers'" perceptions of their needs and the resources available, the judgments of other professionals and the nature of the care relationships that exist. All of these factors are an integral part of any future "package of care" drawn from a combination of people's personal networks and the available voluntary and professional services.

3.18   Most people enter residential care because of their social
        circumstances, not just as a result of their individual
        characteristics. A major thrust behind the community care reforms
        is the acknowledgment that the majority of people currently
        entering residential care do not want to be there and that many
        could have been maintained in their own homes with a
        relatively small amount of additional support from others (Neil
        et al, 1988; Shaw and Walton, 1979; Stapleton, 1976; Townsend,
        1962; Willcocks et al, 1982). Residents are generally not more
        dependent on others for help with self care tasks than many
        living in the community (Bebbington and Tong, 1986; Bowling and
        Bleatham, 1982; Booth et al, 1983; Neil et al, 1988; Wade et al,
        1983). Housing, and particularly the retention of the person's own
        home is a crucial factor in precipitating admissions and
        permanent placement (Neil et al, 1988; Townsend, 1962). Most
        people entering residential care were not receiving intensive
        packages of services that might have kept them at home (Avon,
        1980; Neil et al, 1988), and as many as half of the applicants
        admitted from the community were not receiving home help
        (Neil et al, 1988). In the opinion of social workers, between a
        third and a half of residents could have been kept at home,
        given adequate support (Avon, 1980; Neil et al, 1988).

3.19   It is difficult to imagine that elderly members of the royal
        family will ever need "residential care"; they are able to
        construct their own "package" to maintain themselves in their
        own homes.

3.20   It is also true that children who enter care do so, like the
        elderly, because of their social circumstances, and not just because
        of their individual characteristics. For example, two of the main
        findings of recent research on placements of children in care are
        that:

        "The level of family discord and fragmentation which is
        reported indicates that practical services alone will often be
        insufficient and help with family relationships may be
        essential for effective preventive services.

        "The availability of functioning family and social networks
        seems to be a critical determinant of the need for admission
        and thus a necessary focus for preventive work". (DoH, 1990b)

3.21   Social services professionals will have to act as agents of change
        in social situations as well as gatekeepers of resources. Not all
        social services work is aimed at unmet need. A significant

proportion is directed at the **way** that needs are being met, or not met by other people, in the status quo. Social services and social workers are often involved because somebody has defined existing relationships as a problem: either because they are harmful to participants, as in the case of neglected or abused children; or because a situation leads kin, neighbours or professionals to identify the risk to a person concerned as "unacceptable", for example the isolation of some elderly people; or because their behaviour causes risks to themselves or others as in some mental illness referrals; or because a person's behaviour is defined as deviant if not actually delinquent. All these situations involve several people. Typically, beside the "client" and referrer stand family, friends, neighbours and others who, for many different reasons, share concern as carers and/or victims of the person's behaviour and circumstances.

3.22 The role of the social worker or care manager is not automatically that of direct carer or service provider. It is often **not** necessary for professionals to become an integral part of the process of meeting "client" needs. Their role can be that of an outsider, a broker who links those with needs to those who have the resources to meet them, or "change agent" where intervention is required to modify people's behaviour. The targets of change may be the person whose behaviour is causing concern, the victim of such behaviour or those people whose actions, or lack of them, lead to people continuing to have unmet needs of the kind covered by the Acts. Workers attempting to bring about such change often need to maintain a degree of "marginality", not always appropriate for someone who is an integral part of a caring network (Smale and Tuson, 1989; Smale et al, 1993).

3.23 The roles of professionals in social work and social care can be reformulated to fulfil the bridging functions necessary to provide choice from a coherent set of options. These will include the assessment, negotiation, change agent, care management, "team" development and maintenance functions involved in the co-ordination of services and the social care planning activities required at the local level to provide the bricks of community care and child care services plans.

3.24 In attempting to reform community care and child protection there is a constant danger that effort will be undermined by the basic assumptions that persist about the nature of the problems we are confronting. Many still see all problems in individual terms, and not in terms of all, or even some, of the people who are part of the problem. We keep overlooking what it means to call them "social" services departments and acting as if they were really "individual" services departments; the enterprise is "individual care at home" rather than "community" care. Individualised intervention is not changed by prefixing titles with the much abused, and now almost totally discredited word, "community".

3.25   Ironically, choices are not widened by concentrating on individuals and their internal or physical condition, but by developing different options for their needs to be met, which means enabling them and their carers to enter into negotiations with, and so have some choice between, the different **people** who could meet those needs. If we are to maintain the integrity of "community" care, "social" services and "social" work, we have to confront the constant tendency that we all have to **regress to the individualisation of social problems.**

What is a social problem?

3.26   These issues rest on understanding what constitutes a **social problem**, as distinct from an individual's physical, emotional or psychological problems. People have many different problems, the causes located in many different aspects of their own attributes, their environment or in the interaction between the two. These "causes" are not often known in a strictly scientific sense. These individual problems become a **social** problem when they involve others: when others become concerned either for the person or as victims of their behaviour, or when a person's needs cannot be met by people in the immediate social circumstances of the person and people feel they should be. Thus a frail, elderly person having difficulty preparing their own food, fearful of being alone and without somebody with whom they can share their depression about their physical condition, clearly has "problems". Some may say these problems are an inevitable "fact of life": a feature of "ageing". For this person to be referred to a social services or social work agency or in some other way to be identified as a **"social problem"** is as much a comment on **how their problems are or are not being met by others**, as it is a reflection of the person themselves. To focus on them and their needs alone is not only to ignore potential sources of support, the normal resources called on in these circumstances; but also to misunderstand the very nature of the **social problem** presented by these situations.

3.27   Social services and other professionals using this approach stand little chance of producing positive change in the people's situations they have been called upon to help. They will depend on negotiating for state resources to help such people, and essentially take responsibility for these problems on to themselves as representatives of the state. This is a valid and vital option for many service users and carers. But it is far from the only option, and when used routinely it compounds the social services tendency to "clientise" all who ask or are referred for help, and as in the case of residential care inappropriately to draw into the net people who need not and do not want to make demands on very scarce resources. We should recognise that **social problems are the malfunctioning of a network of people**. The network may be composed of family, friends or neighbours, or other members of the wider community, or the "problem" may be that there are none, or too few, of these people. We have underlined the fact that the vast majority of people's needs are met by carers in the community, without professional intervention. People's needs only become a "social problem" when they are not met. Being old is not a serious problem any more than being a baby is one. Being either, without having appropriate relationships with others is, however, a "social problem" (Smale et al, 1988).

General comments on the process of change

3.28   A basic assumption of the reforms to be implemented through the 1989 Children Act and the 1990 NHS and Community Care Act is the requirement to match social services and social work practice to the problems defined by users, carers and parents, and the needs and resources available in the areas they live in. New ways of delivering services, and of social work intervention, will have to be worked out through partnerships between users, other citizens and professionals from a range of agencies. There can be no universal blueprints for services if consumers are to be involved in their planning and given more choice. For the aims of the acts to be realised the creation of new ways of working and the adaptation of appropriate services developed elsewhere have to become major features of social services and social work organisations.

3.29   As the Griffiths report stated:

"The aim must be to provide structure and resources to support the initiatives, the innovation and the commitment at local level and to allow them to flourish; to encourage the success stories in one area to become the commonplace of achievement everywhere else." (Griffiths, 1988 p.iv)

3.30   Evidence based on the Community Care and Children Acts Implementation Programme at NISW, in which over sixty social services departments participated, showed that many senior managers seemed intent on reorganisations as a primary means of achieving the proposed changes in practice and in their relationship with the public and other service providers. For many, in the absence of any other strategy, this appears to be the only choice for achieving change. If this is true of the general situation, the intention of the reforms "to support the initiatives, the innovation and the commitment at local level and to allow them to flourish" is in serious danger of being pushed aside.

3.31   The tendency to approach all change through structures and procedures means that the centre retains control of the process and content of work and attempts to control outcome. However, the spirit of these reforms is intended to work in the opposite direction: ". . . delegating responsibility for decision-making to the local level wherever possible" (House of Commons, 1989 p.4).

3.32   There is an urgent need to develop a greater understanding of the processes of innovation in practice methods and how these relate to the management of social services departments and other social work agencies. To generate and guide the changes required by the Acts in social services management and social work practice, it is essential that we increase our understanding of the skills and knowledge required and the capacity of those who act as agents of change in their agencies.

3.33   The National Institute for Social Work's Practice and Development Exchange has focused on the diffusion of innovations in several areas and it is clear from this work that many managers are unaware of the need to support innovation in their aepartments, or of how to manage change provoked by social policy initiatives. These issues are being addressed through a Department of Health funded project which began in April 1991 (Smale, 1992).

3.34   Understanding how change is implemented is crucial: evidence from research and development work supports the view that changes in practice and attitudes take place over years, not months, and reorganisations may demoralise and sidetrack workers and management rather than help them to develop practice and services. A machine can be restructured and reorganised at will, and if the engineer knows his or her business, made more efficient and effective. But organisations are not like this; managers do not have the empirical science and hard technological knowledge to inform their redesigns. Organisations, like organisms, change shape as parts of them grow and develop. The most suitable form is determined by its appropriateness and compatibility with its contemporary environment: not the successful completion of a plan drawn up in a previous age.

"Informal" care and statutory services: the need to develop resources

Packages of care can only be put together if human and other resources are available

3.35   "Normal" care is provided by family, friends, neighbours. What constitutes normal care is part of our cultures and so will certainly vary between ethnic groups, from community to community and in different families. "Normal" patterns of care are also influenced by class, race, gender, ethnicity, religion and income levels and the ability to purchase care. Whatever the culture, when immediate families and friends are unable to cope it is naive to assume the "natural" existence of wider networks that can be called upon to meet people's needs without resources being put in to change the way people and organisations are currently relating to each other and to develop the potential for more care and appropriate control in the community. Activities that require developmental resources include:

- intervention to change the relationships in family and immediate networks where the "burden" of care falls on one instead of several carers: enabling users to understand how they can contribute to the family network and others to share care are essential **parts** of caring for the carers;

- the development of schemes to cater for the needs of particular groups of people;

- the development of partnerships between users, both carers and clients, voluntary groups and statutory agencies within the community;

- the formation of partnerships between statutory services and self-help groups to develop and sustain such groups;

- collaboration between workers in different agencies and the development of three-way reciprocal partnerships between agencies and the public they serve.

3.36 Social networks are not only sources of support: they are also sources of conflict, and the location of "social problems"; enabling "normal" care to take place often requires a change in the way people relate to each other in their social networks and not just the delivery of a service (Abrams in Bulmer, 1986; Smale et al, 1988; Gibbons, 1990).

3.37 "Informal" care, the unfortunate phrase used to refer to the care provided by non-professionals, does not come from nothing. Although it is normal for people to be cared for by relatives, friends and neighbours, there are always limits to the care that is currently available (Bulmer, 1986; Sinclair et al, 1988; Sinclair et al, 1990).

3.38 Much has been written about the so-called informal sector and the use of natural helping networks. Advocates of patch-based community social work set great store on the value of developing social networks and the "interweaving" of formal and informal care (Bayley et al, 1985; Hadley and McGrath, 1984). On the other hand critics have drawn attention to the limitations of the care available in social networks (Bulmer, 1987; Finch and Groves, 1983).

3.39 Recent research has differentiated between the kinds of care that are acceptable to those in need and provided by close personal relatives or professionals, for example bathing, and the support that is offered by neighbours and other members of the community, for example occasional shopping (Sinclair et al, 1988). In our view this differing evidence is not necessarily contradictory but reflects the many different variables that exist in disparate neighbourhoods and cultures.

3.40 Practitioners and managers engaged in the development of community based practice in many different parts of Britain have underlined the differences that exist from area to area and the need to develop services accordingly (Smale et al, 1988). They have pointed out that it is crucial that managers and practitioners engage in significant work at the local level if the resources are to be available to expand care in the community for all age groups. Arguing for the need to recognise that social services professionals are required to act as agents of change and not just as resource brokers and deliverers of service, they say:

> "The untapped resources in communities and networks are often talked of as if they were similar to the reservoirs of oil under the seabed. All we have to do to develop these resources is to locate the oil and build a pipeline to areas of need, thus providing 'support' . . . 'The community' is not just a solution— 'the community' has created these problems in the first place. These 'resources'—these potential network helpers—are currently busy doing other things. Formal helpers are working in the old ways; so are the semi-formal helpers, that is, organised volunteers. 'Potential helpers', be they next-door neighbours or relatives, are busy with their own lives . . . There is no evidence to suggest that there are queues of people sitting in a social vacuum waiting to help". (Smale et al, 1988 pp.117–8)

3.41   The development of resources involves intervention designed to change the level of care available in the community. The "market" may provide financially viable facilities, but even when budgets are made available to purchase services, many activities will still need to be undertaken by statutory departments or voluntary organisations fulfilling their innovatory role. There is a potentially enormous bill for care if purchasing care is to replace the motivations that currently underpin the bulk of care in the community, and at the same time ensure the quality of much of the care provided by professionals.

3.42   These activities require staff time. Research conclusions indicate that the time is most likely to be available if specialist workers and managers are appointed within geographically located teams that can collectively maximise essential local knowledge— a theme we return to below. Research and development experience underlines the crucial importance of **workload** management schemes that recognise the vital nature of work beyond caseload management. This is also essential for workers to be able to contribute to community (social) care planning. We have referred above to the need for participative management and the devolution of decisions about resources, and expand on the place of specialist skills and knowledge below.

3.43　Most of the teams who were represented in the Community Social Work Exchange networks had to develop workload management systems that recognised the work that staff engaged in beyond their casework and direct service provision functions. Without such systems indirect work, often referred to as "non-statutory" work, was often a casualty of the pressure of child care referrals, compounded by orthodox assumptions that individual casework was the only, or at least a necessary, response. In contrast to this, three of the teams whose work is described in *Pictures of Practice* (Volumes One and Two) turned to indirect, community orientated work because they found that they did not have the resources to confront high levels of child abuse referrals with orthodox casework alone (Eastham in Darvill and Smale, 1990; Green in Smale and Bennett, 1989; Law in Smale and Bennett, 1989).

3.44　However, many departments still only recognise client numbers as an indication of need. We have often come across teams who have been threatened with or had staff taken from them, when they have been successful in reducing the numbers of children on statutory orders. If this crude approach to the measurement of need and work persists in the new community care planning processes, then the reality of "need" and the provision of resources will be further divorced from each other.

3.45　The Kent community care project and its successors found that there was a danger of care managers working well with individual cases, but not addressing issues that affect all clients in the team. Allocation of resources to activities at this level is essential, as is management recognition that these activities are fundamental and need support. These conclusions are confirmed by Crosbie and Vickery (1989). They found that favourable procedures and practices that facilitated the development of schemes included the vision of managers; a workload management system that not only took account of work other than casework but protected allocated time as "sacrosanct"; the completion of an area needs assessment exercise; and the payment of overtime or time off in lieu.

3.46　Good self-help and collaboration between groups and professional services often improves the care that people and their carers receive, but the evidence suggests that it increases, and does not replace, the demand for public services.

Black and ethnic minority communities: exemplars of care and the need for changed relationships with service providers

3.47   There is opportunity to learn from Black and ethnic minorities and a need to redress the imbalance that exists in service provision. In the introduction we drew attention to the "triple jeopardy" experienced by Black people (Norman, 1985). Greatly improved communication is needed and variety in the provision of services for children and adults is required. These should arise from genuine links between statutory, voluntary agencies and user representatives and local people rather than tokenistic gestures made for short term political ends.

3.48   Many Black and ethnic minority people have turned to others in their own community for care, because it was natural to do so but also because they have been excluded from, or inappropriately catered for, by services of local authorities and voluntary organisations. Strengths have been developed that in some situations demonstrate alternative forms of community care and so ways in which greater choice can be offered to all those who need help.

3.49   But these processes have also led to the perpetuation of significant problems, specifically the over-representation of Black people in the control, as opposed to care, aspects of the system: for example, relatively high proportions of Black children in residential care and the juvenile justice system and lack of access to adult services such as home help. If these disadvantages are not to be perpetuated then non-exploitative partnerships between existing community resources and professional services have to be initiated to overcome the barriers that have often led to Black and ethnic minority people not receiving the services they are entitled to.

3.50   The communication of knowledge and information are crucial dimensions of choice and empowerment. Particular tactics need to be adopted such as undertaking outreach work in places frequented by Black and ethnic minority people to inform them about services. Language can be a barrier which excludes people. People need to be addressed in their own language, simple and jargon-free. This is true for all people irrespective of race, colour or cultural background, but the relationships between orthodox service providers and minority groups has often highlighted the difficulties that exist in most relationships in a more subtle form. There is a growing awareness that attempts to overcome the barriers that exist between Black and white people and professionals can demonstrate how communication between workers and the public can be improved.

3.51   Particular issues are raised for collaboration with Black and ethnic minority community groups. Contracts with voluntary and community organisations will have to safeguard the interests of minority groups through consultation with local communities. The history of consultation with Black and ethnic minority people means that trust has yet to be established in the intentions of social services departments and other agencies. There are problems to be overcome in these relationships: how, for example, will a small, local, voluntary organisation be able to maintain its advocacy role if it bids for a contract to supply services for its constituents?

Assessment and care management: one process, two activities?

3.52   A fundamental problem for care managers, assessors and resource allocators lies in achieving a balance between considerations of **equity** and of more **creative forms of justice**. Here resources are increased in accordance with the individual's personal experience of the need or suffering or the position of particularly disadvantaged groups in society. Targeting has difficulties associated with it; it may tend to favour "creative" justice at the expense of public equity. It will run into even more perverse difficulty if it is based on administrators' or professionals' definitions of the intensity of need rather than on definitions negotiated even-handedly with the service user. A moral balance has to be achieved between these two approaches to justice; this is most likely to be accomplished if the assessment made by care managers is **both** user responsive **and** is seen to be accountable also to **both** organisational **and** professional perspectives of priority and justice.

3.53   We have stressed that social problems are the malfunctioning of a network of people and that the network may be composed of family, friends or neighbours, or other members of the wider community. Often the "problem" is that there are too few of these people in the dependent person's environment.

3.54   In such situations there is no simple way of identifying the needs or demands of service users. There is often inevitable conflict between the demands and needs of referrers, such as medical professionals, carers and dependent people, that is between the different "users" of services, and between other people in the "client's" family and wider network. To arrive at and maintain a workable and good enough package of care as defined by all these users, the role of those undertaking assessments and care management will revolve around negotiation. They will have to negotiate an assessment and way of managing the problem within all the above conflicting needs, attitudes, expectations and definitions of the "problem" and its "solutions".

3.55   Awareness and appropriate action in working with ethnic minorities in the community should increase workers' awareness of the complexity of all communication between people from different backgrounds and in different roles. To develop services that are sensitive to the idiosyncratic cultural and subcultural needs of different people will require workers to develop communication skills and strategies to find out how people define their problems and their potential solutions within their particular circumstances.

3.56   The different perceptions of the problem that inevitably exist complicate any evaluation of the services provided. This is further complicated by the social control issues that are present, in a more or less explicit way, in most social situations requiring intervention.

3.57   The views of all the people in the existing and potential networks will be crucial to "an assessment" of what is needed. Collecting them will be the first step in getting these people to work together as the team, that is the "package of care". A **team** in this sense is used to mean people who depend on each other to some extent to carry out tasks or to get their work done.

3.58   Each person in the social network will have their own perception of "the problem", and opinions of what needs to be done, based on what they have been doing and could do to support the person at home. This will often include both "client" and "carers" and others who do or might help, such as relatives, friends, neighbours, and other professionals including the GP, district nurse, occupational therapist, home care organiser, and so on. These perceptions will be influenced by their beliefs and expectations and formed by their cultural background, personal experience and, in the case of the professionals, their training and conditioning by their organisation's procedures, norms and values. These influences will also affect the professionals' expectations of the people they work with and they will need to develop their awareness of the need to understand people from different cultures without slipping into, and so perpetuating stereotyping. To do this it is necessary for them to use and develop their knowledge and skills, specifically their ability to empathise with a wide range of people and to maintain an appropriate marginality (Smale and Tuson, 1988; see Smale et al, 1993 for models of assessments and definitions of skills.)

3.59   In the development work reviewed and much of the practice studied by researchers, the distinctions made by service providers between different activities, "client" groups and professionals, made little sense to users and other members of the public. The emphasis is on relationships with people beyond the individual "client" to assess "need" and mobilise support, and the practical reality of "care packaging" being about negotiating who will and can do what to help. These factors lead us to question the wisdom of a simple split between assessment and care management.

3.60   The assessment of child care situations is a complex process and rightly subject to statutory reviews in acknowledgement of the inevitability of change and the dangers of intervention being based on obsolete perceptions and decisions about individuals and their situation. Any person's circumstances can change with remarkable speed and assuming that workers are in touch, precipitate quick decisions about changes in practice and service delivery. But we know that this has not always happened and that children have sometimes "drifted" or even been "lost in care" (DoH, 1985; Packman, 1986).

3.61   The circumstances were often characterised by a split between the "assessor", typically the field social work staff, and the "service providers", those providing residential or foster care. The system of "key workers" was introduced to maintain a constant link with the child and to make sure of the current relevance of the responses to the child's needs and changes in the social situation. The intention is that the care manager system will have many of the same functions, monitoring changes in circumstances; the assessment and reassessment a constant feature of the work. An "assessor" may carry out the initial review of a social situation and collect the opinions of people at the time of referral but this is only the start of a service provider's involvement in a continuous process. The people who are parts of any subsequent "package of care" will quite rightly make their own assessments of the needs of the various people involved including themselves and their own contribution. The heart of the care manager's role is gathering and responding to these changing assessments.

3.62   Care management is the "co-ordination" of different people's efforts, and where appropriate, budgetary control. It involves initiating, maintaining and monitoring the effectiveness of a team of people composed of all the people in the situation. It will often require working with people to adjust their behaviour in terms of what they contribute and how they do it. Care managers will constantly be reassessing and listening to the reassessments of members of the team as the social situation inevitably changes over time. It is not "just management" in a narrow administrative sense, and is more than planning services and allocating and controlling resources. In practice many of the resources used in community care and the protection of children are controlled by ordinary members of the public and other organisations or determined by central government through social security benefits and so beyond the authority of any "care manager".

The flexibility, sensitivity and variability of "care packages"

3.63   **A package of care is not like a basket of goods and services; it is actually a fluid set of human relationships and arrangements.** The care manager's main task will be to make the efforts of the people involved coherent; to make sure that the care of a dependent person is not dropped like the baton of a badly co-ordinated relay team. **Teamwork between these people is essential and the care manager's role will focus on team development and maintenance.**

3.64   The evidence suggests that people want different elements of their care carried out by different people. The Networks project, for example, found that many elderly people wanted personal care to be carried out by a paid person if no close relative was available and not by neighbours, who were however often considered to be acceptable for befriending and action in an emergency. The different cultural norms that exist over these matters in different communities and ethnic groups and individuals' idiosyncratic preferences within them will have to

be taken into consideration if a user sensitive service is to be
provided.

3.65   What is perhaps more important than an awareness of these
        variations is the fact that these generalisations are only
        generalisations. What a person wants, what they and their
        carers expect and want from services has to be discovered and
        negotiated by workers. To form partnerships with people,
        workers will need to be sensitive to the almost infinite
        variability that exists. Tailor-made solutions have to become the
        norm. At best, off the peg solutions fit by chance. At worst, they
        cause grave offence and cause minority groups to be deprived of
        services altogether. We know that people from ethnic minorities
        are under-represented in the take up of services provided by SSDs
        and other community care agencies. We also know that they tend
        to be over-represented amongst those involved in the social
        control functions of the same agencies (Black Perspectives
        Exchange, 1990). These facts highlight the need for services to be
        more sensitive to all their actual and potential users and the
        need for workers and managers to develop the vital skills
        required to communicate effectively with all citizens and,
        especially, users.

3.66   David Challis expressed the view in discussions with us that
        there need to be variable care management schemes providing a
        continuum, from autonomy of a person providing their own care
        management, through to situations where a person has their own
        care manager to cater for very complex needs requiring long-term
        care.

3.67   The community based projects and area teams reported on all
        placed great store on the provision of informal responses to
        people's problems and ready access to services by workers based
        as locally as possible to increase their accessibility to the public
        and their knowledge of and partnerships with other local sources
        of support. The flexibility of these projects will need to be
        adopted by the mainstream of social services provision if
        "flexible, sensitive" services are to become commonplace. These
        services were provided by social services department teams or
        voluntary organisation projects acting with local people. In our
        discussions some concern was expressed by researchers that the
        introduction of the machinery of contracting may make the
        response of service providers slower and too inflexible to meet the
        ever changing nature of people's day to day relationships.

3.68   The overlap with contract management adds further complexity to flexible and effective care management. This overlap underlines the need to treat aspects of assessment and care management as being located at different points on a continuum. One way this continuum is already manifesting itself is in the emergence of two stages of assessment, one carried out by the social services department and the other by the providing agency, for example a residential home or resource such as a Crossroads Care Attendant scheme. The statutory care manager identifies priority "clients" and allocates the level of budget, but then hands over responsibility for the detailed assessment and ongoing reviews and reassessments to the provider, who is contracted accordingly. A key aspect of the care manager's role thereafter is to monitor and evaluate compliance with the contract. It should be recognised that monitoring the continuing relevance of the contract involves further assessment independent of the service provider.

Local knowledge: the building blocks of "social" care planning

3.69   There is a danger that thinking and planning for the implementation of the Community Care and Children Acts reforms are split from each other. From the NISW experience of working with managers engaged in planning the implementation of the two Acts a possible unintended consequence of the two sets of guidelines is that many departments seem to be following the separate "form" of the proposals. The early Community Care documents were published with green covers while the Children Act publications were in red; many departments have set up separate planning processes to work on these guidelines, as if they have a "red" and a "green" set of implementation problems to solve. Some are reorganising into children and adult divisions, rather than following the explicit recommendation, the **"content"** of the proposals, which stresses:

> "The two programmes are consistent and complementary and, taken together, set a fresh agenda and new challenges for the social services authorities for the next decade. There is no intention of creating a division between child care and community care services; the full range of social services authority functions should continue to form a coherent whole." (House of Commons, 1989 Chapter 1, p.3, para 1.3).

One planning process is required to develop a coherent strategic plan and appropriate allocation of resources for all user groups.

3.70 This policy was confirmed in a speech by Sir William Utting:

"I do not seek to minimise the differences between the Children Act and community care; but there are principles, needs and services in common which support the continuing desirability of combining them within the same organisational framework." (Utting, 1991)

3.71 Some departments are including services for children in their community care planning processes. This enables them to balance needs and resources across the whole of their responsibilities thus minimising competition between different client groups. Community based practice teams have demonstrated that this approach to "social care planning" can lead to the mobilisation of community resources and the commissioning of services for the benefit of both groups.

3.72 Social care plans should be built from the bottom up based on the aggregate of local knowledge gained through partnerships with local people, assessments and the experience of negotiating packages of care. We have stressed that vital information is known only to those in direct contact with service users, their supporters and other potential or actual community resources. For social care plans to be genuine, information about the needs and resources that exist within a geographical community, or in and around a "community of interest" (those people related to each other through involvement with a shared problem or interest) is essential: they have to be built up from this knowledge of what exists.

3.73 Like the number of words in a Shakespeare play, the number of people in any particular category in a community is of little significance on its own. The number of one kind relative to another is of more, but perhaps only academic, interest. But just as it is the sound and meaning of words as they are woven into the complex pattern of language that matters, so how people actually relate to each other and the juxtaposition of their different needs, expectations, beliefs and behaviour is of crucial importance.

3.74 The language of community or social care plans should be accessible to the majority of people. Community care plans should not only be based on local knowledge, but also need to be built up in partnership with local people, through communication with them in language that they understand. The participation in the planning and operation of social services of local people from all the different groups who make up our multi-cultural society and of the different users who call on social services is still a new frontier. Continued development work as well as persistence will be required to maintain new attitudes in the face of existing organisational habits and planning systems that are administratively more convenient.

Targeting services to those who need only a little intervention

3.75   The allocation of services to those who need relatively small amounts of support, or linking these people to resources in the community, is vital to maintaining many people in their own homes, to "care for the carers", and to implementing one of the "key components of community care (which) should be: services that intervene no more than is necessary to foster independence" (House of Commons, 1989 p.5).

3.76   Statements such as the following peppered our consultations with those involved with this research:

> "The success of the community care reforms is dependent upon how departments will cope with the bulk of those needing support".

> "You should make services available to people when **they** need them and not when a crisis has been reached."

3.77   The research is clear: a little help is of enormous significance, whether to individuals living at home or carers struggling to maintain others in the community. Fears were expressed that the targeting of services could mean that those people who needed such relatively small inputs could be left with nothing.

3.78   The screening of referrals for assessment and "packages of care" could develop into a situation analogous to "community alternatives to custody". The acceleration of people "up the tariff" would not work in quite the same way, but there is a serious danger that services will **only** be available to those who might otherwise incur the costs of residential care. Practitioners are aware of those situations where it is necessary to emphasise a person's problems to release resources and conscious that sometimes "clients" feel forced to "lay it on" to get what they need. Nothing will contribute more to the stigmatisation of "clients" than the need to exaggerate problems.

3.79 Access to services as a normal way of tackling normal problems, and information of what is available to whom, are key issues in the process of "intervening as little as possible to foster independence". Projects that have **taken** this position as central to their philosophy are described in *Pictures of Practice* (Henderson's and Macfarlane's contributions in Smale and Bennett, 1989).

3.80 It must be remembered that the "most needy" are often the same people as those who "need a little or nothing" at a different point in time. Drawing on the experience of innovatory managers and practitioners who had developed community based services the authors wrote in *Community Social Work: A Paradigm for Change*:

> "Making a service available to a few, 'the most needy', may save resources in the short term, but only at the expense of those who receive those services and, in the long run, those who pay. To qualify people must satisfy certain criteria, or to put it another way, justify the label. Receiving the service then confirms that label. Such an approach perpetuates stigmatisation, and the web of reciprocal behaviour involved may then hold such people in their situations more firmly than straightforward material dependency upon the service (Smale, 1984). Selective services concentrated on 'the most needy' also fail to prevent those not yet in the category from arriving at that point. Such people are often caught in a spiral of escalating unmet needs as their problems compound and exacerbate each other, since help is withheld until their situation is bad enough to demand it.

> "The cost of services to 'the most needy' is typically extremely high since they are, by definition, beyond the point where relatively small amounts can be spent, in either time or material resources, to maintain a potentially deteriorating position. In these ways direct service to the few often causes more resources to be spent on the few than might have been spent more effectively on indirect, preventative strategies targeted on a wider group of people." (Smale et al, 1988)

3.81 To intervene no more than is necessary to foster independence is to intervene **early**. To concentrate only on those with the greater needs is to intervene **late**. It is vital that resources are targeted on the large numbers of people who are being supported by carers in the community if the reforms are going to "maintain adults and children at home, in their family, or in their familiar community for as long as possible", support carers, and "intervene no more than is necessary to foster independence".

Management implications in achieving effective collaboration

3.82 Partnerships with users, community groups, and other agencies at a local level requires a high degree of **participative management** within the agency for two major reasons:

- **First:** the delegation of appropriate responsibility to workers forming partnerships with local people. If workers are to empower people, politicians and senior management have to empower them to make decisions at the local level, in collaboration with "clients", their carers and other people in the community.

- **Second:** all those in the work-force with local knowledge, or specialist group knowledge of user needs and demands and available resources, should be involved in contributing this information to the formulation and implementation of departmental policy, plans and practice.

3.83 Devolved resource management is crucial; evidence from the Kent Community Care Scheme, research on services for elderly people (Sinclair et al, 1990), the development of schemes for all client groups (Crosbie and Vickery, 1989), and Gibbons' (1990) work on services to families, all stress that the people with the most knowledge of local circumstances and users' lives need to be involved in, and not continue to be removed from, resource allocation.

3.84 In their extensive review of research on services for the elderly, Sinclair and his colleagues (1990) note that collaboration does not work on a grand scale between agencies, and managers would be better focusing their energy and attention on specific areas of work where achievable goals can be set. Gibbons (1990) has joined a continuing line of researchers who have found that joint planning between organisations at a senior level is not reflected at local level. Local collaboration needs to be seen as an area of development through negotiation in its own right. Professional and management attention has to be devoted to these activities and time allocated to these tasks in workload management systems.

Specialist staff in locally-based teams and needs-led community based services

3.85   We have drawn attention to the dangers of restructuring the organisation as the prime means of implementing the proposed reforms. The status quo must not be retained but the process of change is crucial. If users of services are to be effectively consulted this should be an integral part of, rather than follow, reorganisation. Successful organisations are normally in a constant state of flux as they innovate to stay relevant to their changing circumstances (Kanter, 1984; Peters, 1988; Smale, 1992). As practice changes through the developing partnerships that workers and managers form with people in the community so we anticipate that the organisation will evolve in its internal relationships, that is, restructuring will take place.

3.86   A corollary of user-led services is a practice-led organisation. The place of specialist workers within the organisation will vary according to the demands of the area. But certain generalisations can be made to maintain consistency with the assumptions of the reforms.

3.87   There is little evidence that relates different organisational structures to the outcomes of services (Challis and Firlie, 1987). Summarising the main findings on policies, planning and decision-making in child care, and their implications for practice, it is concluded that:

> "Studies of various departmental structures have reinforced the message that reorganisation may solve some problems but usually creates others and there is no blueprint suitable for all types of authority. Improvements in practice are not likely to result from further organisational change." (DoH, 1990b p.75)

The research reviewed supports small locally-based generalist area teams and services, with specialists within them, rather than centralised services provided through specialist divisions based on administrative categories of "clients". The evidence does not suggest that the "fresh agenda and new challenges for the social services authorities for the next decade" is a return to the pre-Seebohm pattern of organisation of the 1950s, even if the "departments" have a single directorate.

3.88   On the other hand specialist workers need to work with others in their own specialism to develop knowledge, skills and agency policies. Thus a matrix of geographically based and specialist worker teams needs to be organised within the agency.

3.89   Such a matrix is common in other organisations which have specialist workers, for example personnel officers, production engineers, stock handlers and a wide range of craft specialists, each of whom is responsible to a geographically-based line management responsible for the "team" working together to achieve their tasks. But each person is also accountable to a functional manager; for example, personnel staff will be accountable to the personnel director for the implementation of the organisation's policy in this specialist field.

3.90   Research supports devolved resource management and decentralised decision-making. Challis and his colleagues have demonstrated the value of "case managers" holding their own budgets and also the need for them to develop their teamwork to address area needs (1986; 1990). The research and development work on community-based practice emphasises the significance of local access for increasing choice through the expansion of the range of services available to and from local people (Bayley, 1989; Hadley, 1984; Hadley and McGrath, 1984; Hadley et al, 1987; Seyd et al, 1984; Smale and Bennett, 1989; Darvill and Smale, 1990). The research also has implications for the place of specialisation in departments.

3.91   Specialisation within SSDs and other social work and social services agencies is required for staff:

   ●   to form effective links with local voluntary organisations;

   ●   to promote schemes and community based projects;

   ●   to develop the practice expertise of social workers and other key staff (Gibbons, 1990; Crosbie and Vickery, 1989; Sinclair et al, 1990).

3.92   But the way this is done and the level at which it is done is crucial. It is necessary to acquire and maintain an intimate knowledge of local networks and to build relationships and partnerships with local people and resources. The evidence indicates that the vital information is typically known by those staff who, while in direct contact with users, are also often removed from decisions about resource allocation: staff including home-helps, occupational therapists, social work assistants and social workers. This knowledge needs to be pooled and used to plan services and resource allocation at a local level, and to be passed up to the directorate as the building blocks of social care planning.

3.93   The combined efforts of these staff need to add up to a coherent single service for the users who do not (nor should they be expected to) divide their problems up in ways that are convenient for service providers.

3.94   Choice depends upon information and the availability of services. Geographical location is crucial to access to, and knowledge of, services. The transport difficulties experienced by people trying to use services should not be underestimated. This is not just a rural problem. In many major cities and small towns practitioners and managers attempting to extend access to services experienced significant problems related to the availability of appropriate transport.

3.95   Although specialisation is often not desirable at the first point of contact between the public and the agency which needs to be local and accessible, or even for initial assessments, specialisation is highly desirable at the second stage of assessment when arrangements for care or intervention are being negotiated. There is evidence that this helps workers and managers to build effective inter-organisational networks of voluntary/community/self-help groups who identify with a particular issue, area of need or "client" group (Crosbie and Vickery, 1989; Gibbons, 1990).

3.96   When responsibility for provision has been passed by the social services department to voluntary, community, or independent organisations they can build their own multi-professional paid staff teams, unconstrained by traditional public service boundaries.

3.97   The successful implementation of the reforms will depend upon **"team development"** at different levels within agencies and across agency boundaries. We have already drawn attention to the fact that a successful "package of care" is in practice a team of people. The division of labour involved in specialisation requires good **teamwork** if coherent services are to be established and maintained and the needs of the people in user networks are to be "managed" and not dropped as they pass from one person to another.

3.98   Geographically-based teams can achieve this mix of specialism and coherence. Specialist teams or divisions, however, will make the dovetailing of services more difficult at the interface between the department and the public. It is acknowledged that it may be administratively more convenient to divide departments in this way, but we assume that the overriding principles are that services should be "needs-led" and coherent, rather than designed for the convenience of service providers. Departments have to be able to demonstrate collaboration of a high order **internally** as well as with other people and organisations in the community.

3.99   A review of the skills required to carry out community based practice through teamwork at all levels led the authors to argue for a radical rethinking of the nature and location of social work training (Smale and Tuson, 1988).

3.100   The Griffiths report and *Caring for People* were clear in their recommendations for decentralised services with devolved budgets and decision making. Griffiths' recommendations made clear the intention that managers should foster local initiatives and motivation, and capitalise on innovation:

>   "The aim must be to provide structure and resources to support the initiatives, the innovation and the commitment at local level and to allow them to flourish; to encourage the success stories in one area to become the commonplace of achievement everywhere else. To prescribe from the centre will be to shrivel the varied pattern of local activity." (Griffiths, 1988 p.iv)

3.101   When we set up Practice and Development Exchange at the National Institute for Social Work in 1983, a major task of developing community based practice was seen as mainstreaming the innovation that was taking place in certain projects that appeared to be making progress in implementing many of the values that have been adopted by the new policies. These projects' characteristics included:

- implementing values such as the development of partnerships between professionals and citizens and between agencies;

- increasing the range of options open to people and so increasing choice;

- making services more available through easier access;

- expanding the role of social service personnel beyond the direct provision of care to individuals;

- the planning of services and practice based on area profiles of local needs and resources, attempts to extend user choice and control;

- fostering independence and supporting carers by developing support throughout people's social networks and through locally based schemes and self-help groups.

3.102   By 1990 the aim of mainstreaming such innovations had been turned on its head. In the conclusion to *Pictures of Practice II* we wrote:

> "In our view it is necessary for all social services and social work activities to take on more of the characteristics of special projects. Special projects typically have to justify the work that they are going to do based on an assessment of needs and resources, justifying their staffing levels on the work required, and being explicit about how their methods of work will tackle the problems presented to them. The whole exercise is time limited and costed, the project managed so as to stay within both constraints, and the consequences of action evaluated." (Smale and Tuson, 1990 p.163)

3.103   A major lesson is that dynamic, innovatory teams need to have the kind of independence and autonomy associated with special project status. For the changes in practice involved in implementing the reforms to become more widespread, more of the mainstream social services tasks need to be handled through teamwork geared to the characteristics of such projects. This is not to argue that existing organisations should or can become one big "special project", but that social work and social services should increasingly be characterised by a proliferation of such projects and teams. The resources expended on attempting to achieve and sustain uniformity and perpetuating large monolithic bureaucracies could be used to foster the growth of smaller, relatively autonomous teams, closer to the consumer and more immediately responsive to changes in the problems to be tackled.

Such teams would have to enter into many partnerships with similar teams and other organisations, but the need for these partnerships would arise from the problems being addressed, rather than from remote bureaucratic assumptions and blueprints.

3.104 The implementation of the reforms will require **team development** with citizens and "professionals", at all levels within agencies and across organisational boundaries. Teamwork skills should be central to professional training and education.

Some final thoughts: an expression of pessimism founded on optimism

3.105 The authors of *The Kaleidoscope of Care* warn us that properly managed social services and social work departments, voluntary organisations and private agencies and good practice in the caring professions are a necessary but insufficient response to the challenges of community care for elderly people. They argue that the right housing and income maintenance policies and adequate resources for social services are also crucial if people are to live independently (Sinclair et al, 1990). Access to buildings, public transport and employment will be as crucial for the empowerment of other people as appropriate educational opportunities and pre-school provision and day-care facilities are for children and their parents.

3.106 Increasing attendance, disability and invalid care allowances and carers' premium so that people can buy their own "care packages" would increase empowerment. Information about available services is also crucial to choice, or even the basic recognition of the existence of any alternative between a carer struggling on and residential care.

3.107 Access is a crucial dimension of the ability to obtain a service: paying for what you can get is another. But not all aspects of care can be bought.

3.108 The sad conclusion in a few years' time may be that community care for all age groups will have been tried and will have failed, whereas in fact it will have been advocated, partially implemented, tested a little, but largely fragmented by competing priorities. These stem from the urge to save money spent on residential care, the assumption that good packages of care can be bought and the belief that an expansion of the private sector will lead to better care in the community.

3.109   The community care reforms and the Children Act, this review, and much of the thinking during the 1980s about community based practice and service delivery is based on an awareness of the fact that the bulk of care is carried out in the community by relatives, friends and neighbours, sometimes referred to as "informal care".

3.110   A major fault in implementing the current reforms may prove to be a failure to build on people's normal capacity to care by overlooking the fact that carers and cared for can be given more support and choice by encouraging the involvement of a wider section of the community.

3.111   Financial incentives are not at the heart of normal care in the community. Indeed it costs many people much to fulfil these roles. The practitioners, managers and researchers whose work is reviewed here would not advocate that these people should be exploited, rather that the care of "dependent" people is a normal process made vulnerable by the fact that all too often it is shared by too few people. This normal way of meeting people's needs should be promoted so that the "burden" of care is shared with more people. The capacity of the community to care should be extended, and not replaced, by services whether public or private.

3.112   Currently the absence of carers, the discovery of inappropriate or delinquent behaviour, a breakdown in caring arrangements or the overstretching of these resources by increased dependency is all too often dealt with by a complete change of gear. The formal services either resist involvement for lack of resources, or at the point of crisis, take over.

3.113   The normal way for our community to care when the normal systems break down is to attempt to buy an alternative. This is the same response as sending food to famine-stricken people, essential for immediate survival, but a short-sighted and extremely expensive long-term solution. There is a need to put in resources at times of crisis but these will not account for long-term care. This can only be provided by changes in patterns of care over time: by long-term development work.

3.114   This form of intervention has been tried in relatively isolated places, tested a little, and is now supported by major policy proposals, but many of its complexities are being overtaken by the current rush to set up new "mechanisms" for purchasing and providing community care services, and to implement new statutory powers under the Children Act. Griffiths proposed the establishment of mechanisms for putting Barclay into practice (para 27, p. vii). It is crucial that we do not lose sight of what the "machine" is designed to help us produce, or the fact that it produces nothing without partnerships with a wide range of citizens and professionals.

3.115   This is **not** an argument for reducing the role of public services nor is it a prescription for cheap community care. It is an argument for improving the care of people by directing professional time, expertise and energy at developing people's resources in the community. These recommendations are not revolutionary but their implementation has yet to take place on a wide scale. This work has been going on over the last few years and there is experience and expertise to be built on and much more work to be done to develop management and practice further.

3.116   We all need to be cared for in the community. All people are dependent upon others for different aspects of their care at various stages in their lives and nearly all people will be called upon to provide it: six million people do not constitute a small minority. Normally people will be cared for by their relatives, with a few supported by friends, neighbours and public services. Private and public services are crucial supplements to this care and vital for many who have no real alternative. A major over-simplification is to see those who receive formally organised care as different categories of people rather than recognise that they are people at a particular stage in their lives whose "needs" are not met by those around them.

3.117   The unmet needs of a "dependent person" are as much a statement about the availability of these people as they are of the "dependency needs" of the individual. It makes sense then to put resources into this half of the problem and not to put all our effort into professional services from either the public, voluntary or private sectors; not just to target the "most needy" but also those social situations where care is most absent.

References

[References with an asterisk are those which were reviewed in this study; those without an asterisk are additional documents cited]

Abraham, F. and Webb, B. (1989) *Mental Health and Self-Help Support.* COVAS Occasional Paper no. 5. London: Tavistock Institute.

Abrams, M. (1978) *Beyond Three-Score and Ten: A First Report on a Survey of the Elderly.* Mitcham: Age Concern.

Abrams, P., Abrams, S., Humphrey, R. and Snaith, R. (1981) *Action for Care: A Review of Good Neighbour Schemes.* Berkhamsted: Volunteer Centre.

* Ahmad, A. (1990) *Practice with Care.* London: Race Equality Unit, National Institute for Social Work.

* Ahmad, B. (1990) *Black Perspectives in Social Work.* Birmingham: Venture Press for Race Equality Unit, National Institute for Social Work.

Avon (1980) *Admissions to Homes for the Elderly: A Survey of Alternatives.* Bath: Avon County Council Social Services Department. (Unpublished.)

Barclay Report (1982) *Social Workers: Their Role and Tasks.* London: Bedford Square Press.

* Bayley, M., Seyd, R. and Tennant, A. (1989) *Local Health and Welfare.* London: Allen and Unwin.

Bebbington, A. and Miles, J. (1989) The background of children who enter local authority care. *British Journal of Social Work,* 19 (5).

Bebbington, A. and Tong, M. (1986) Trends and changes in old people's homes: provision over twenty years. In Judge, K. and Sinclair, I. (eds) *Residential Care for Elderly People*. London: HMSO.

* Black Perspectives Exchange (1990) *Surviving in White Organisations*. London: Practice and Development Exchange, National Institute for Social Work.

Booth, T. A., Barritt, S., Berry S., Martin, D. N. and Melotte, C. (1983) Dependency in residential homes for the elderly. *Social Policy and Administration*, 17 (1) pp. 46–62.

Bowling, A. C. and Bleathman, C. (1982) The need for nursing and other skilled care in local authority residential homes for the elderly. Research report no. 5: overall findings and recommendations. *Clearing House for Local Authority Social Services Research*, (9), pp. 1–65.

Brocklehurst, J.C. and Tucker, J.S. (1980) *Progress in Geriatric Day Care*. London: King Edward's Hospital Fund for London.

* Bulmer, M. (1986) *Neighbours: The Work of Philip Abrams*. Cambridge: Cambridge University Press.

Carey, K. (1986) *Leaving Care*. Oxford: Blackwell.

* Challis, D. and Davies, B. (1986) *Case Management in Community Care*. Aldershot: Gower.

Challis, D. and Firlie, E. (1987) Changing patterns of fieldwork organisation: the team leaders' view. *British Journal of Social Work*, 17, pp. 147–167.

* Challis, D., Chessum, R., Chesterman, J., Luckett, R. and Traske,K. (1990) *Case Management in Social and Health Care*. Canterbury: University of Kent Personal Social Services Research Unit.

Chisholm, I. and Fletcher, P. (1979) *The Park Club: A Study of a Club Run by Voluntary Effort to Help Support Confused Elderly People and Their Families*. Aylesbury: Buckinghamshire County Council Social Services Department.

*   Crosbie, D. and Vickery, A. (1989) *Community Based Schemes in Area Offices*. Report to the Department of Health. London: National Institute for Social Work.

*   Crosbie, D., Bennett, W., Smale, G. and Waterson, J. (1989) *Disseminating Community Social Work in Scotland*. London: National Institute for Social Work.

*   Darvill, G. and Smale, G. (eds.) (1990) *Partners in Empowerment: Networks of Innovation in Social Work*. Pictures of Practice Volume II. London: National Institute for Social Work.

Department of Health (1989) *An Introduction to the Children Act 1989: A New Framework for the Care and Upbringing of Children*. London: HMSO.

Department of Health Social Services Inspectorate (1989) *The Care of Children: Principles and Practice in Regulations and Guidance*. London: HMSO.

Department of Health (1990a) *Community Care in the Next Decade and Beyond: Policy Guidance*. London: HMSO.

Department of Health (1990b) *Patterns and Outcomes in Child Placement: Messages from Current Research and Their Implications*. London: HMSO.

Department of Health (1991) *Working Together Under the Children Act 1989: A Guide to Arrangements for Inter-Agency Co-operation for the Protection of Children from Abuse*. Children Act Consultation Paper No. 22. London: HMSO.

Department of Health and Social Security (1985) *Social Work Decisions in Child Care: Recent Research Findings and Their Implications*. London: HMSO.

*   Dutt, R. and Ahmad, A. (1991) Griffiths and the Black persective. *Social Work and Social Sciences Review*, 2(1), pp.37–44.

Edwards, C. and Carter, J. (1980) *The Data of Day Care*. London: National Institute for Social Work.

Finch, J. and Groves, D. (1983) *Labour of Love*. London: Routledge and Kegan Paul.

Flynn, N. and Miller, L. (1991) *Caring in Our Communities: The Management Agenda.* Briefing Paper 4. London: National Institute for Social Work Information Service.

* Gibbons, J. (1990) *Family Support and Prevention: Studies in Local Areas.* London: HMSO for National Institute for Social Work.

Graham, H. (1984) *Women, Health and the Family.* Hemel Hempstead: Wheatsheaf.

Green, H. (1988) *Informal Carers: General Household Survey, 1985.* London: HMSO.

Griffiths, R. (1988) *Community Care: Agenda for Action. A Report to the Secretary of State for Social Services.* London: HMSO.

* Hadley, R. and McGrath, M. (1984) *When Social Services are Local: The Normanton Experience.* London: Allen and Unwin.

Hadley, R., Webb, A. and Farrell, C. (1975) *Across the Generations.* London: Allen and Unwin.

Hadley, R., Dale, P. and Sills, P. (1984) *Decentralising Social Services: A Model for Change.* London: Bedford Square Press.

Hadley, R., Cooper, M., Dale, P. and Stacy, G. (1987) *A Community Social Worker's Handbook.* London: Tavistock.

Hatch, S. (1978) *Voluntary Work: A Report of a Survey.* Berkhamsted: Volunteer Centre.

* Hatch, S. and Hinton, T. (1986) *Self-Help in Practice: A Study of Contact a Family.* Sheffield: *Community Care*/University of Sheffield Monographs.

Hatch, S. and Mocroft, I. (1970) Factors affecting the location of voluntary organisation branches. *Policy and Politics,* 6.

Hatch, S., Mocroft, I. and Smolka, G. (1981) *Social Services Departments and the Community: Report to the Department of Health and Social Security.* (Unpublished.)

Hearn, B. and Thomson, B. (1987) *Developing Community Social Work in Teams: A Manual for Practice*. London: National Institute for Social Work.

Holme, A. and Maizels, J. (1978) *Social Workers and Volunteers*. London: British Association of Social Workers/Allen and Unwin.

House of Commons (1989) *Caring for People: Community Care in the Next Decade and Beyond*. Cm 849. London: HMSO.

* Jones, A. (1991) *Black Community Care: Report of the Black Communities Care Project*. Leeds: National Institute for Social Work.

Kanter, R. Moss (1984) *The Change Masters: Corporate Entrepreneurs at Work*. London: Allen and Unwin.

Kelly, G. *Patterns of Care: Child Care Careers and the Patterns that Shape Them*. Belfast: DHSS Northern Ireland. (Unpublished.)

Leat, D. (1979) *Limited Liability? A Report on Some Good Neighbour Schemes*. Berkhamsted: Volunteer Centre.

Leat, D. (1983) *A Home from Home*? Mitcham: Age Concern Research Unit.

Leat, D., Smolka, G. and Unell, J. (1981) *Voluntary and Statutory Collaboration: Rhetoric or Reality?* London: Bedford Square Press.

Leat, D., Tester, S. and Unell, J. (1986) *A Price Worth Paying? A Study of the Effects of Government Grant Aid to Voluntary Organisations*. London: Policy Studies Institute.

* Levin, E., Sinclair, I. and Gorbach, P. (1983) *The Supporters of Confused Elderly People at Home*. Report to the Department of Health and Social Security. London: National Institute for Social Work Research Unit.

* Levin, E., Sinclair, I. and Gorbach, P. (1989) *Families, Services and Confusion in Old Age*. Aldershot: Avebury.

Macdonald, A.J.D. et al (1982) An attempt to determine the impact of four types of care upon the elderly in London by the study of matched groups. *Psychological Medicine*, 12 (1).

* Manuel, P. (1991) *Black Communities Care: Information About Your Rights*. Leeds: National Institute for Social Work.

Mendel, J. (1979a) Confusion unconfounded. *Community Care*, 16 August, pp.19–20.

Mendel, J. (1979b) *Report to Family and Community Services (Sheffield Social Services Department) on MIND's Woodhouse Project*. (Unpublished.)

Miller, C., Crosbie, D. and Vickery, A. (1991) *Everyday Community Care: A Manual for Managers*. London: National Institute for Social Work.

Moore, J. and Green, J.M. (1985) The contribution of voluntary organisations to the support of caring relatives. *Quarterly Journal of Social Affairs*, 1 (2).

Neill, J., Sinclair, I., Gorbach, P. and Williams, J. (1988) *A Need for Care? Elderly Applicants for Local Authority Homes*. Aldershot: Avebury.

Norman, A. (1985) *Triple Jeopardy: Growing Old in a Second Homeland*. Policy Studies in Ageing No. 3. London: Centre for Policy on Ageing.

Packman, J., Randall, J. and Jacques, N. (1986) *Who Needs Care? Social Work Decisions about Children*. Oxford: Blackwell.

Parker, G. (1985) *With Due Care and Attention: A Review of Research on Informal Care*. Occasional Paper no. 2. London: Family Policy Studies Centre.

Peters, T. (1988) *Thriving on Chaos: Handbook for a Management Revolution*. London: Macmillan.

Power, M. (1979) *The Use of Volunteers in the Home Care of the Very Old*. Report to the Department of Health and Social Security. (Unpublished.)

*   Richardson, A. (1983) *Self Help and Social Care: Mutual Aid Organisations in Practice.* London: Policy Studies Institute.

•   Sainsbury, E. (1990) *The Work of the Community Social Work Exchange, National Institute for Social Work.* Report to the Department of Health. (Unpublished.)

Seebohm, F. (Chairman) (1968) *Report of the Committee on Local Authority and Allied Personal Social Services.* Cmnd. 3703. London: HMSO.

*   Seyd, R., Tennant, A., Bayley, M. and Parker, P. (1984) *Community Social Work.* Sheffield: University of Sheffield.

Shaw, I. and Walton, R. (1979) Transition to residence in homes for the elderly. In Harris, D. and Hyland, J. (eds) *Rights in Residence.* London: Residential Care Association.

Shenfield, B. and Allen, I. (1972) *The Organisation of Voluntary Service: A Study of Domiciliary Visiting of the Elderly by Volunteers.* London: Policy and Economic Planning.

*   Sinclair, I., Crosbie, D., O'Conner, P., Stanforth, L. and Vickery, A. (1988) *Bridging Two Worlds: Social Work and the Elderly Living Alone.* Aldershot: Avebury.

*   Sinclair, I., Parker, R., Leat, D. and Williams, J. (1990) *The Kaleidoscope of Care: A Review of Research in Welfare Provision for Elderly People.* London: HMSO for National Institute for Social Work.

Smale, G. (1991) *Innovations and Change in Practice: The Work of Practice and Development Exchange, National Institute for Social Work.* (Unpublished.)

*   Smale, G. and Bennett, W. (1989) *Pictures of Practice Volume I: Community Social Work in Scotland.* London: National Institute for Social Work.

*   Smale, G. and Tuson, G. (1988) *Learning for Change.* London: National Institute for Social Work.

*   Smale, G., Tuson, G., Cooper, M., Wardle, M. and Crosbie, D. (1988) *Community Social Work: A Paradigm for Change.* London: National Institute for Social Work.

* Smale, G. and Tuson, G. with Biehal, N. and Marsh, P. (1993) *Empowerment, Assessment, Care Management and the Skilled Worker*. London: HMSO for National Institute for Social Work.

Smale, G. (1992) *Managing Change Through Innovation: Toward a Model for Developing and Reforming Social Work Practice and Social Services Delivery*. Report to the Department of Health Social Services Inspectorate. London: Practice and Development Exchange, National Institute for Social Work.

Sokolovsky, J. (1989) Bringing culture back home: ethnicity, ageing and family support. In Sokolovsky, J. (ed) *The Cultural Context of Ageing: Global Perspectives*. Westport: Berdin and Garvey.

* Sommerlad, E. and Webb, B. (1988) *Survey of Self-Help Support Projects*. London: Tavistock Institute.

Stapleton, B. (1976) *A Survey of the Waiting List for Places in Newham's Hostels for the Elderly*. London: London Borough of Newham Applied Research Section.

Stein, M. and Carey, K. (1986) *Leaving Care*. Oxford: Blackwell.

Tennant, H. and Bayley, M. (1985) The eighth decade: family structure and support networks in the community. In Yoder, J.A. et al (eds) *Support Networks in a Caring Community*. Dordecht: Martinus Nijhoff.

Tinker, A. (1984) *Staying at Home: Helping Elderly People*. London: HMSO.

Townsend, P. (1962) *The Last Refuge*. London: Routledge and Kegan Paul.

Utting W. (1991) The shape of things to come. *Community Care* Conference *Shaping a New World*, Boston, 12th April 1991. (Unpublished.)

Vallender, I. (1990) Family centres—who needs them? *Concern* (74).

* Van der Eyken, W. (1982) *Home-Start: A Four-Year Evaluation*. Leicester: Home-Start Consultancy.

Vincent, J. (1986) *Constraints on the Stability and Longevity of Self-Help Groups in the Field of Health Care*. Loughborough: Loughborough University Centre for Research in Social Policy.

Wade, B., Sawyer, L. and Bell, S. (1983) *Dependency with Dignity*. London: Bedford Square Press.

Wedge, P. (1989) *Social Work: A Fourth Look at Social Work into Practice*. Birmingham: British Association of Social Workers.

Wedge, S. *Growing Up Alone: Final Report*. (Unpublished.)

Willcocks, D., Peace, S., Kellaher, L. and Ring, J. (1982) *The Residential Life of Old People: A Study in 100 Local Authority Homes*. Survey Research Unit Research reports nos. 12, 13. London: Polytechnic of North London School of Applied Social Studies and Sociology.

Printed in the United Kingdom for HMSO.
Dd.0297603, 7/94, C50, 3396/4, 5673, 265224.